Promoting the Well-Being of the Critical Care Nurse

Editor

SUSAN BARTOS

CRITICAL CARE NURSING CLINICS OF NORTH AMERICA

www.ccnursing.theclinics.com

Consulting Editor
CYNTHIA BAUTISTA

September 2020 • Volume 32 • Number 3

ELSEVIER

1600 John F. Kennedy Boulevard • Suite 1800 • Philadelphia, Pennsylvania, 19103-2899

http://www.theclinics.com

CRITICAL CARE NURSING CLINICS OF NORTH AMERICA Volume 32, Number 3
September 2020 ISSN 0899-5885, ISBN-13: 978-0-323-76060-7

Editor: Kerry Holland
Developmental Editor: Laura Fisher

Critical Care Nursing Clinics of North America (ISSN 0899-5885) is published quarterly by Elsevier Inc., 360 Park Avenue South, New York, NY 10010-1710. Months of issue are March, June, September, and December. Business and Editorial Offices: 1600 John F. Kennedy Blvd., Suite 1800, Philadelphia, PA 19103-2899. Periodicals postage paid at New York, NY and additional mailing offices. Subscription prices are $160.00 per year for US individuals, $428.00 per year for US institutions, $100.00 per year for US students and residents, $206.00 per year for Canadian individuals, $538.00 per year for Canadian institutions, $230.00 per year for international individuals, $538.00 per year for international institutions, $115.00 per year for international students/residents and $100.00 per year for Canadian students/residents. To receive student/resident rate, orders must be accompanied by name of affiliated institution, data of term, and the *signature* of program/residency coordinator on institution letterhead. Orders will be billed at individual rate until proof of status is received. Foreign air speed delivery is included in all *Clinics* subscription prices. All prices are subject to change without notice. **POSTMASTER:** Send address changes to *Critical Care Nursing Clinics of North America*, Elsevier Health Sciences Division, Subscription Customer Service, 3251 Riverport Lane, Maryland Heights, MO 63043. **Customer Service: 1-800-654-2452 (US and Canada); 314-447-8871 (outside US and Canada). Fax: 314-447-8029. E-mail:** JournalsCustomerService-usa@elsevier.com **(for print support) and** JournalsOnlineSupport-usa@elsevier.com **(for online support).**

Reprints. For copies of 100 or more of articles in this publication, please contact the Commercial Reprints Department, Elsevier Inc., 360 Park Avenue South, New York, New York, 10010-1710; Tel.: 212-633-3874, Fax: 212-633-3820, and E-mail: reprints@elsevier.com.

Critical Care Nursing Clinics of North America is covered in *MEDLINE/PubMed (Index Medicus), International Nursing Index, Nursing Citation Index, Cumulative Index to Nursing and Allied Health Literature, and RNdex Top 100.*

Contributors

CONSULTING EDITOR

CYNTHIA BAUTISTA, PhD, APRN, FNCS, FCNS
Associate Professor, Egan School of Nursing and Health Studies, Fairfield University, Fairfield, Connecticut, USA

EDITOR

SUSAN BARTOS, PhD, RN, CCRN
Assistant Professor of Nursing, Egan School of Nursing and Health Studies, Fairfield University, Fairfield, Connecticut, USA

AUTHORS

CATHERINE ALVAREZ, MA, BS, RN, CNML, HNB-BC, PCCN
Professional Development Specialist, Yale New Haven Hospital, New Haven, Connecticut, USA

SUSAN BARTOS, PhD, RN, CCRN
Assistant Professor of Nursing, Egan School of Nursing and Health Studies, Fairfield University, Fairfield, Connecticut, USA

AUDREY M. BEAUVAIS, DNP, MSN, MBA, RN
Associate Professor, Egan School of Nursing and Health Studies, Fairfield University, Fairfield, Connecticut, USA

ROBERT L. BOGUE, BS
President, Thor Projects LLC, Carmel, Indiana, USA

TERRI L. BOGUE, MSN, RN, PCNS-BC
Chief Operating Officer, Thor Projects LLC, Carmel, Indiana, USA

BRENDA BURSCH, PhD
Professor of Clinical Psychiatry and Biobehavioral Sciences and Pediatrics, David Geffen School of Medicine at UCLA, Los Angeles, California, USA

DEENA KELLY COSTA, PhD, RN
Assistant Professor, Co-director, National Clinician Scholars Program, School of Nursing, The Institute for Healthcare Policy and Innovation, University of Michigan, Ann Arbor, Michigan, USA

ALYSSA ERIKSON, PhD, RN
Associate Professor, Nursing, California State University, Monterey, California, USA

LEE A. GALUSKA, PhD, RN
Adjunct Assistant Professor, UCLA School of Nursing, Executive Director, Center for Nursing Excellence, UCLA Health, Los Angeles, California, USA

JIN JUN, PhD, RN
Post-Doctoral Research Fellow, National Clinician Scholar, School of Nursing, The Institute for Healthcare Policy and Innovation, University of Michigan, Ann Arbor, Michigan, USA

JENNIFER L. McADAM, PhD, RN
Associate Professor, Nursing, Samuel Merritt University, Oakland, California, USA

DEBORAH McELLIGOTT, DNP, ANP-BC, AHN-BC, HWNC-BC, CDE
Nurse Practitioner, Center for Wellness and Integrative Medicine, Katz Institute for Women's Health, Northwell Health, Roslyn, New York, USA; Faculty, International Nurse Coach Association, North Miami, Florida, USA; Clinical Assistant Professor, Donald and Barbara Zucker School of Medicine at Hofstra/Northwell, Uniondale, New York, USA

ANNA M. RODRIGUEZ, BSN, RN, PCCN, CCRN
Registered Nurse, Endoscopy, University of Utah Health, Salt Lake City, Utah, USA

LINDA NANCY RONEY, EdD, RN-BC, CPEN, CNE
Associate Professor, Egan School of Nursing and Health Studies, Fairfield University, Fairfield, Connecticut, USA

KAREN STUTZER, PhD, RN
Associate Professor, Nursing, The College of Saint Elizabeth, Morristown, New Jersey, USA; Mentor, Thomas Edison State University, Trenton, New Jersey, USA

JOANNE TURNIER, DNP, RN, ACNS-BC, HN-BC, HWNC-BC
Adjunct Instructor, Department of Nursing, St Joseph's College, Patchogue, New York, USA; Adult Clinical Nurse Specialist, Faculty, International Nurse Coach Association, Health and Wellness Nurse Coach, Center for Wellness and Integrative Medicine, Roslyn, New York, USA

Contents

> Healthy nurses are essential for optimizing population health, patient care experiences, and health care cost-efficiency. Critical care nurses are at increased risk of developing physical and psychological symptoms due to their high-stress work environment and exposure to traumatic events. There is growing recognition for the value of implementing nurse-centered, team-based, and organizational-wide levels of intervention designed to mitigate the impact of high work stress and trauma on health professionals. The central assertion of this article is that meaning and joy in nursing practice are contributors to professional well-being and part of the solution for achieving the quadruple aim.

> Intensive care unit (ICU) nurses report some of the highest levels of stress and burnout because they are exposed to excessive workloads, end-of-life concerns, prolonged care, and ethical dilemmas. Supporting ICU staff through self-care and mindfulness programs is successful in improving stress and burnout and in promoting resilience. Addressing barriers to engaging in self-care practices and identifying unit-specific needs are important to consider when implementing wellness programs. Micro-restorative practices can alleviate immediate stress generated from patient care and provide a moment of peace in busy ICUs. Leadership and organizational support are vital in identifying the need for and promoting wellness programs.

> Ethically challenging situations are an increasing phenomenon in the nurse's environment, and literature on the subject is growing. Morally challenging experiences common in the critical care environment include end-of-life situations, barriers to providing the best care possible, and lack of organizational resources. These experiences can lead to moral distress and subsequent negative impacts on the clinician. Emerging in the literature are strategies to address the impact of moral distress through the development of moral resilience. Moral resilience is gained through personal commitment and organizational support.

Burnout—a combination of emotional exhaustion, depersonalization, and a diminished sense of individual accomplishment—is a serious issue for critical care nurses. Burnout has been examined as an individual's emotional state, but burnout is also a social phenomenon that may spread among colleagues through emotional contagion. Current interventions to reduce burnout are either person directed or organization directed; few interventions focus on the critical care nursing team and their social support and interactions. This article reviews burnout in critical care nursing through the lens of emotional contagion. We offer suggestions for team-based interventions to address burnout in critical care nurses.

Academicians who maintain a critical care clinical practice encounter numerous stressors, especially during the COVID-19 pandemic, which can influence well-being. This article provides historical perspectives on the stressors inherent in working in the critical care environment as well as the stressors of working in the academic environment. It proposes the application of the synergy model as a framework to help improve the well-being of academicians who practice and teach critical care. The most valuable strategy to improve professional well-being is for organizations to take a systems approach. The article focuses on approaches that are potentially within each individual's control.

Critical care nurses frequently provide end-of-life and bereavement care. This type of care is rewarding, but can put nurses at risk for moral distress, compassion fatigue, and burnout. By incorporating self-care into their routine, critical care nurses minimize this risk and maintain their own health and well-being. This article provides suggestions for promoting physical, emotional, and spiritual self-care for nurses caring for dying intensive care unit patients and their families. A case scenario illustrates the importance of this concept. Practical examples of self-care are highlighted along with discussion on how leadership can support self-care and maintain a healthy work environment.

The need for self-care in critical care nurses is recognized on a national level. Stress, unhealthy lifestyles, and chronic disease in the general population is mirrored in nursing, affecting burnout, retention, quality outcomes, and well-being. Integrative approaches to promote well-being are supported by nursing theories and tools such as the Integrative Health and Wellness Assessment (IHWA). Through coaching techniques and the IHWA, nurses can support their self-development via self-assessment, self-reflection, self-evaluation, and self-care. This article discusses the role of the IHWA and a coaching process to aid critical care nurses in implementing sustainable self-care strategies.

Burnout is reaching epidemic levels among health care providers. It negatively impacts individual providers, the care team, facility, and patients. Increased employee turnover, job dissatisfaction, and conflict are found whenever staff becomes burned out. Patient outcomes and satisfaction are negatively impacted. Although burnout is increasing in health care, much can be done to change the level of burnout and improve employee satisfaction. Individuals can learn the factors that lead to burnout and specific actions that can help prevent and recover from burnout. This information can be used to transform health care and decrease burnout and its effects.

Art in nursing is present in various forms and there is ample literature exploring creativity, including journaling for clinicians, intensive care unit diaries for patients and providers, and music therapy for patients. Illness narratives, depictions of the sick, or the effects of disease are commonly represented in media. This article highlights how creativity and various mediums of artistic expressions may can be used as a self-care practice and aid in boosting empathy in health care providers. Theories on empathy are presented as well as selected representations of nursing as creative expressions and the importance of promoting creativity and empathy.

Promoting the Well-Being of the Critical Care Nurse

CRITICAL CARE NURSING
CLINICS OF NORTH AMERICA

SERIES OF RELATED INTEREST

Nursing Clinics of North America
http://www.nursing.theclinics.com

THE CLINICS ARE AVAILABLE ONLINE!
Access your subscription at:
www.theclinics.com

Preface

The Juxtaposition of Caring

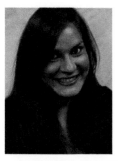

Susan Bartos, PhD, RN, CCRN
Editor

Nursing sits at the juxtaposition of self-care. On one side is the career: the call of nursing: absolute and definitive selflessness. Nursing is the ability, skill, and desire to care for another being during a time of need and desperate vulnerability. On the other side is the insatiable, self-motivated hunger for more: more knowledge, more technology, more validation, and faster, more evidence-based advancement. The fast-paced, intense environment is magnified in the critical care unit and for those who practice within the environment. The constant push and pull are exhausting: it's tiring, it's stressful, and it burns us out.

This issue of *Critical Care Nursing Clinics of North America* was curated at a pivotal time. The well-being of the critical care clinician was a topic of interest a year ago, at the time this issue was envisioned; however, this topic has morphed into a vital necessity. Many of these titles were written pre-COVID-19, yet the fundamental messages of decreasing stress, enhancing moral resilience, coping with bereavement, and supporting those clinicians who may be practicing in multiple environments, such as inpatient and in an academic institution, are perhaps even more applicable now. Within these pages is the guiding wisdom to find the restoration of purpose, to flourish through creativity, and to finding joy in caring for the critically ill.

In the current climate of health care, a strong foundation of wellness is essential for critical care clinicians. Mental clarity, strength, happiness and joy, gratitude, perspective, and tenacity surround the foundational pillars of a critical care nurse who is guided by evidence-based practices. Multifaced wellness programs, self-restorative practices, and solidifying wholesome purpose for critical care nurses can lead to longevity in the career while promoting safer patient outcomes and initiatives. Imagine a world where the 2 sides of the juxtaposition are not under constant opposing stress, but

Crit Care Nurs Clin N Am 32 (2020) ix–x
https://doi.org/10.1016/j.cnc.2020.06.001
0899-5885/20/© 2020 Published by Elsevier Inc.

ccnursing.theclinics.com

are connected and balanced. Imagine living in peace, not as patients, not as nurses, but as people.

Susan Bartos, PhD, RN, CCRN
Egan School of Nursing and Health Studies
Fairfield University
1073 North Benson Road
Fairfield, CT 06824, USA

E-mail address:
sbartos@fairfield.edu

Meaning, Joy, and Critical Care Nurse Well-Being
A Call to Action

Lee A. Galuska, PhD, RN[a],*, Brenda Bursch, PhD[b]

KEYWORDS

- Quadruple aim • Critical care nurses • Burnout • Meaning and joy

KEY POINTS

- Healthy nurses are essential for optimizing population health, patient care experiences, and health care cost-efficiency.
- Critical care nurses are at increased risk of developing physical and psychological symptoms due to their high-stress work environment and exposure to traumatic events.
- There is growing recognition for the value of implementing nurse-centered, team-based, and organizational-wide levels of intervention designed to mitigate the impact of high work stress and trauma on health professionals.
- Validated assessment approaches, evidence-based interventions and support resources, and organizational commitment are key features of a successful approach for achieving the quadruple aim.
- Meaning and joy in nursing practice are contributors to professional well-being and part of the solution for achieving the quadruple aim.

With clinician burnout occurring in as many as 54% of nurses and physicians in the United States, clinician well-being has been commanding increasing attention.[1] Healthy professionals are essential to achieving the triple aim for health care transformation as described by Berwick and colleagues. They claimed that this transformation would only occur through the simultaneous pursuit of 3 aims: improved population health, better patient care experiences, and cost reduction in our health care system.[2] In 2015, a fourth aim of improving the experience of providing care was recommended in acknowledgment of the vital role of caregivers and the importance of promoting clinician well-being and joy in work.[3] The National Academy of Medicine recommends a systems approach to address clinician burnout and promote professional well-being.[1] The recommendations have significant implications for nurses in all settings,

[a] Center for Nursing Excellence, UCLA Health, 924 Westwood Boulevard, Suite 720, Los Angeles, CA 90024, USA; [b] David Geffen School of Medicine at UCLA, 760 Westwood Plaza, Semel 48-241, Los Angeles, CA 90024-1759, USA
* Corresponding author.
E-mail address: LGaluska@mednet.ucla.edu

Crit Care Nurs Clin N Am 32 (2020) 349–367
https://doi.org/10.1016/j.cnc.2020.04.002
0899-5885/20/© 2020 Elsevier Inc. All rights reserved.

ccnursing.theclinics.com

as they embrace their role in health promotion and illness prevention for themselves and their colleagues, as well as the patients they serve. Meaning and joy in nursing practice are contributors to professional well-being and are part of the solution for achieving the quadruple aim.

A FRAMEWORK FOR NURSE WELL-BEING

Martin Seligman, often considered the founder of positive psychology, proposed a well-being framework composed of 5 elements including *positive emotions, engagement, relationships, meaning,* and *accomplishment.*[4(pp14,24)] Seligman created a pneumonic, the PERMA theory of well-being,[4(p16)] to reflect these elements. Each of these measurable elements contributes to well-being but are also pursued for their own sake (without conscious intent to improve well-being).

The goal of the PERMA theory of well-being is human flourishing.[4(p26)] "Well-being is a combination of feeling good as well as actually having meaning, good relationships, and accomplishment."[4(p25)] Each of the elements of the well-being theory, described later, have relevance to nursing practice, implications for nurse well-being, and increase the potential for nurse flourishing for the benefit of the individual, patients, and health care organizations.

Positive Emotions

Positive emotions include happiness, joy, and pleasure that are experienced subjectively by the individual. Positive psychology and the study of joy or happiness have a long history and continue to be of interest as we strive to uncover the keys to satisfaction and success in our personal and professional lives. Popular and business literature, along with scholarly publications, has addressed the value of happiness for individuals, organizational productivity, and the economy.[5–7] Daniel Gilbert described the interest in the study of happiness from many perspectives saying "Psychologists want to understand what people feel, economists want to know what people value, and neuroscientists want to know how people's brains respond to rewards."[7(par3)] In health care, Sikka and colleagues wrote about the importance of clinicians finding joy in their work. They stated, "The core of workforce engagement is the experience of joy and meaning in the work of healthcare. This is not synonymous with happiness, rather that all members of the workforce have a sense of accomplishment and meaning in their contributions."[3(p608)] They emphasized that joy in health care work was essential for improving patient care. In 2017, the Institute for Healthcare Improvement (IHI) proposed a framework for joy in work where they described the impact of the experience of joy on "individual staff engagement and satisfaction, but also patient experience, quality of care, patient safety, and organizational performance" as well as strategies to improve joy in work at the individual, organizational, and system levels.[8(p5)] Joy in the work of health care has been framed as a key driver of clinician well-being and the performance of the health care system.

Engagement

Seligman describes engagement in terms of "flow," when an individual is using all of his or her cognitive and emotional resources in an activity and is completely absorbed in it, even losing track of time.[4(p11)] Csikszentmihalyi also studied flow and its contributions to joy and moments of "optimal experience" characterized by a feeling of purpose and full engagement.[9] Engagement in work draws on individual strengths and one's sense of purpose and is linked to empowerment, job satisfaction, job turnover, and other important organizational outcomes.[10] In nursing, work engagement has been conceptually described as "the dedicated, absorbing, vigorous nursing practice that emerges from settings of autonomy and trust, and results in safer, cost-effective patient outcomes."[11(p1424)] Key drivers and factors contributing to nurse engagement relate to the meaningfulness of the work along with the health and safety of the work environment, including work-life balance and supportive, healthy relationships with managers, nursing, and interprofessional colleagues.[12,13] A focus on engagement strategies has the potential to improve nurse well-being as well as important patient, staff, and organizational outcomes.[10]

Relationships

Having positive relationships is another well-established contributor to well-being. For nurses, this includes therapeutic relationships with patients and their families, healthy collaborative relationships with colleagues, and relationship with self. These 3 key relationships are highlighted in the relationship-based care framework used by many health care organizations to drive person-centered care.[14] For nurses, relational job-characteristics include the opportunity to form relationships with patients and their families, positively affect their lives, and see the difference they make. The psychological impact of these relational job characteristics contributes to nurse personal and professional well-being.[15] True collaboration and healthy, respectful relationships with colleagues are elements of a healthy work environment framework and have been shown to contribute to nurses meaning and joy in their work.[16] Self-care, self-compassion, and self-acceptance have also been shown to contribute to nurse well-being.[17,18] One qualitative study highlighted that nurses sometimes need encouragement ("permission") to be compassionate toward self.[19]

Meaning

Seligman asserts that people "want meaning and purpose in life" and that a meaningful life is about "belonging to and serving something that you believe is bigger than the self."[4(p12)] A sense of meaning and purpose in work have been shown to increase worker engagement and satisfaction, along with improved individual and organizational outcomes.[20,21] For nurses, an opportunity to practice in alignment with their "perceived calling"[22(p828)] contributed to their engagement and satisfaction in their work. The ability to practice in alignment with their own values, identity, and desire to make a difference contributed to meaning and joy.[16] When health care professionals feel that their work matters and that they are making a difference in the lives of others, it strengthens their resilience and reduces their risk of burnout.[23] When they are able to engage in meaningful work at least 20% of the time, they experience less burnout.[24]

Accomplishment

Accomplishment is the fifth element of Seligman's theory based on the belief that the pursuit of success, mastery, and achievement are important to the experience of well-being. Making an impact or difference provides a sense of fulfillment and brings joy and pride. Nurses at all levels and their interprofessional colleagues are constantly striving to improve outcomes for individual patients, communities, and organizations, and this ties to the triple aim of improving the health of populations, the patient experience, and decreasing the cost of health care. Achieving and sustaining excellence in nursing and patient care is the goal of both the Magnet Recognition Program and the American Association of Critical Care Nurses Beacon Award for Excellence Program. High-performing individuals, teams, and organizations are constantly striving for higher levels of achievement and performance excellence. Reaching milestones along the journey to excellence fuels joy, engagement, and well-being.

VALIDATION OF PERMA THEORY OF WELL-BEING AMONG NURSES

Each of the elements of Seligman's well-being theory is interconnected in the lived experience of nurses. Thus, pursuit of nurse well-being, with the goal of nurse flourishing, requires a systems approach with an appreciation for complexity in the work of health care. One of the recommendations for a systems approach to professional well-being includes defining profession-specific fulfillment and well-being.[1] A qualitative study of US nurses in various practice settings and roles (including critical care nurses) aimed to enhance understanding of their experience with meaning and joy and contributing factors.[16] The themes provide insights into experiences that contribute to nurse well-being as described by Seligman[4] and to joy and meaning in health care work as proposed in the quadruple aim by Sikka and colleagues.[3] The study findings reported by Galuska and colleagues included 4 themes and 3 subthemes as described later.

Fulfilling Purpose, "I Am a Nurse"

The theme—Fulfilling purpose, "I am a nurse"—reflected the tendency of study participants to offer their reasons for becoming a nurse.[16(p157)] These reasons included a perceived calling to serve and desire to help others and make a difference. They described a connection with their own values, beliefs, and sense of purpose. In addition, this theme captured the participants' descriptions of the interest in the scientific foundation of nursing as well as the fulfillment that came with caring for others and practicing the art of nursing.

Meaningful Human Connection

"Human connection and relationships enable nurses to provide care that makes a difference, is meaningful, and makes them feel joyful about their impact"[16(p157)] with patients and families as well as interprofessional and nursing colleagues or students.

Impact, the "Wow" Factor

The third theme—Impact, the "wow" factor—represented the powerful experience of seeing the positive impact of their nursing practice on patients, families, or colleagues, which was reported to be a source of joy as well as meaning.[16(p158)] The experience of joy through making a meaningful difference came from multiple sources and validated the contributions that the nurses were making.

The Practice Environment

Galuska and colleagues[16(p159)] reported that "the practice environment and the people in it" were major factors in nurses' ability to experience meaning and joy in their practice. First, the subtheme of teamwork refers to healthy relationships and support from both nursing and interprofessional team members that were described as important in enabling the nurse to have meaningful and joyful experiences. The second subtheme relates to leaders who effectively role model a commitment to nursing, patients, and joy in their leadership practice. "Those who created the conditions for nursing voice, autonomy, and engagement contributed to meaning and joy in nursing practice."[16(p159)] Third, the opportunity to grow and develop to their full potential was meaningful and positive for nurses.

QUOTES FROM STUDY PARTICIPANTS

Secondary analysis of the interview transcripts of critical care nurse study participants was conducted, along with analysis of 2 additional interviews conducted by Galuska, to gain further insights into the experiences of critical care nurses. The quotes by nurses in adult and pediatric critical care settings shared later illustrate the 4 themes.

Fulfilling Purpose, "I Am a nurse"

This theme was reflected in the words of one critical care nurse who said, "I think nursing for me was so much the right decision for me and my own values in life.[16(p157)] Being able to give back to other people and help other people." Another nurse shared, "Part of the joy comes from you go into critical care and emergency medicine when you're—I don't want to call it an adrenaline junky—but you generally thrive in those really high stress environments…"

Nurses were interested in the art and science, the challenge of solving complex problems through critical thinking and experience, mastery of technology, and being a partner in saving lives. For example, one nurse described becoming expert in the use of the Impella device and stated, "There were issues that physicians were bringing to me and asking me about the device and it just felt so awesome! It's like I literally saved a life today! Those are the moments that I think I find such joy."

Meaningful Human Connection

One pediatric intensive care unit (PICU) nurse shared her perspective stating,[16(p157)]

We're just so lucky in our roles because we do see people at their worst, but we get to be a part of it and that's so unusual that you get to experience these really deep meaningful moments with strangers and they accept you and they embrace you and they're grateful for you, most of the time. It's just such an honor to be with these families who are battling and with these kids who are so resilient and so strong and so willing to do whatever it takes for their own life. It just gives you such perspective and it makes you so grateful for your own life…

Another critical care nurse shared this reflection,

Working in the ICU is challenging to say the least. The patients you take care of are critically ill. They're very complex. You're dealing with the patient, but also their family at probably what is the worst time in their life. I think what drives me in that unit and what makes me want to keep coming to work in the morning is those moments I'm able to have with my patient or my family member just finding their humanity because I think it's so easy, especially as our health care system evolves, to become detached from the person that you're caring for, and to really start looking at them in terms of the medications they're on or the disease that they're fighting and I really appreciate those small moments that I'm able to get to know who my patient is, who the family is that's supporting them and that makes it seem all the more worthwhile to me to have that connection with them and maybe impact their life in some way beyond the physical care that I'm providing as a nurse.

Several participants spoke about doing the "little" or "small" things for patients or families as they got to know them and were attuned to their individual needs. One nurse shared this reflection,

Then when I reflect back there are small things. It wasn't major things that I did for the patient. Everything was under control, like hemodynamics or whatever, but I think just the comfort and letting him get a good night's sleep and taking care

of the family… They couldn't thank me enough. I guess that kind of makes it very meaningful coming from them. At the end of the day I said "Okay this was very meaningful achieving their goal. I felt that satisfaction and the meaningful connection with the patient.

As their colleagues in other settings, critical care nurses valued the meaningful connection they made with other nurses and members of the interprofessional team. One nurse stated, "I feel that meaning for me in nursing has really been found in not only my patients, but …in my relationships with my colleagues whether that's nursing, assistant personnel, care partners, physicians…" This nurse went on to share,

I think in the PICU the reason why we had such comradery and such meaningful relationships was that the work was so challenging and it was similar to probably kind of a M.A.S.H. unit or some kind of war zone. The work was so hard that everyone just clung together and took care of each other. …There were times where the meaning came directly from the families – their gratitude and their attention to your attention to detail, your ability to manage all these conflicting priorities. That was very meaningful to be able to tie it all together and care for not only the patients, but the nurses because I think that was huge. To care for one another was huge…. It was our peers that really gave us what we needed and that's why we stuck together. … that kind of Band of Brothers thing that you get in war or even in team sports, you know, when you really rely on each other, it's a good feeling. It makes what you do more meaningful.

IMPACT, THE "WOW" FACTOR

Critical care nurses often used the word "wow"as they described seeing positive outcomes emerging from their practice.[16(p158)] For example, one nurse said, "Wow I really did whatever I could. It's like inner peace that it brings you, that you did all your best that you can do to meet the patient's family needs." Another nurse spoke of the challenges in the ICU environment of not knowing how things worked out for a patient: "ICU is difficult because we don't often see people get well and go home. We see people well enough to leave the ICU, but not to sort of go home and be fully functioning." Another nurse added, "But I always tell people we have really high highs and really low lows, but those high highs really carry you." She and several other nurses spoke of the powerful experience of seeing a patient return to the hospital to visit and thank them after making a full recovery.

I will never forget the day he walked into our unit…. All of a sudden I turned and he's walking and I'm like "He looks so familiar. I think I know him." And it turned out to be the kid that had been essentially levitating out of his bed for months in the PICU and he had made a complete recovery, and he was talking about training for a marathon, and he was back in school, and he was happy. …he remembered the voices of nurses and the presence of nurses and it was just so fulfilling to see this kid make a full recovery after what we had seen for so long.

Sometimes the impact was related to supporting a patient and family through a peaceful death in the ICU. Several participants spoke about it as an honor and privilege to accompany patients and families through this meaningful experience.

When I go and I'm able to enter a really awful situation and still find something positive out of it. It's a type of joy I think, but it's a feeling of peace or calm that I'll leave work with sometimes and I really try and cling onto those and remember those moments because they don't always happen. But after reaching what I think is a meaningful end for a patient and being able to walk with a family with that, I think I finish my shift and I really feel like I did something. I left an impact. They might not remember my name, but I think that they'll remember the interaction that we had.

Nurses also expressed the meaningfulness of having an impact of colleagues. One said, "… it's also a huge thing to hear from a colleague that you made a difference or that they appreciate your impact." One area where nurses believed they were making a significant difference was through difficult times on the unit or through the professional governance structure. One described how she made an impact and felt valued, "…in my professional governance role my colleagues need my input, they need my support, they need me to make the connections for them, connect them with the resources they need. So I think that feeling of being needed, but also being valued." Another nurse shared her impact as a unit council leader stating, "But when things were really tough people were coming to me for guidance and people were coming to me to try to make things better. …blossomed into this opportunity for all of us to bond and to make our unit a better place, and truly to make it better for the patients and the families." She described how positive this experience was and went on to say "…we're just going to riseas one. It's pretty powerful things to be a part of and I feel lucky."

The Practice Environment

Healthy teamwork with nurses and interprofessional colleagues was essential in critical care.[16(p159)] One shared, "I think a huge part for me is just working in an interprofessional team that works well together. That is, a huge element in making the work that we do meaningful and more joyful. It feels really good to have all these different pieces of the puzzle coming together with a common goal just to make our patients' lives better." Nurses described feeling valued, appreciated, supported through effective teamwork. "…it really invigorates that passion that we all started with and…it makes it that much easier to know that I have a good group of people behind me supporting me, also beside me helping me when things get really tough."

Leaders in critical care, in formal leadership roles as well as mentor roles, contribute to the ability of nurses to find meaning and joy in their work. "I think having really good leadership is really important. I think arguably the most important thing is to have leaders who are not only setting a good example and creating a good environment, but also I think it's so important to inspire the staff that you're working with." One nurse spoke to the importance of leaders who take the time to get to know their staff as individuals and provide support for practice experiences that will bring them meaning and joy. Other important leadership activities included providing meaningful recognition to nurses as individuals and celebrating as a team. Facilitating opportunities for nurses to hear positive patient feedback and outcomes also contributed to meaning and joy.

Nurses described the importance of mentors who would provide opportunities for growth and guidance for the journey. One nurse shared,

I also think having really strong mentors and preceptors throughout my career has been important, like having those who you could trust to ask questions of but who could also push you to stretch a little bit further and learn a little bit more and become a little bit more confident. It's those who have that kind of combo pack of great compassion and great competence and are able to navigate the tough waters of taking care of really sick kids in a way that doesn't squash that compassion within themselves but actually somehow they become even more compassionate just because of the need for it.

Critical care nurses, as their colleagues in other settings, described and valued opportunities for formal and informal learning, support for certification, and career advancement. Professional governance councils were described by multiple nurses as a vehicle for learning, gaining perspective, contribution, and growth as clinical leaders. It offered the opportunity to increase engagement and make a difference in the environment and patient care. Nurses described feeling empowered and valued and derived significant meaning and joy from the experience. One nurse captured it this way,

> So I think it kind of all started when Jenny took me under her wing and became an informal mentor to me, and helped me to engage in some activities that we were doing on the unit ... I started just getting a better understanding of all that went on behind the scenes to improve our practice for our patients and our nurses, and the rest of the staff. I just realized that I got so much joy out of trying to make the environment that we worked in healthy and happy and a really nice, warm, and loving environment. So I've over the last few years become more and more engaged in some of our hospital-wide councils and that has been really meaningful and it's really allowed me to see the bigger picture and to understand the struggles that everybody else is experiencing, but also build a camaraderie and really feel connected to other people in the hospital versus just my tiny little unit that's just one piece of the puzzle.

This secondary analysis of critical care nurses' experiences with meaning and joy in their practice affirms that it is possible for critical care nurses to experience all of the necessary elements to promote well-being in their practice. Study participants described positive emotions or joy, engagement, positive relationships, meaningful work, and a sense of accomplishment. Some of the solutions are things they could do as individuals. Other solutions require action at the unit and organizational level. Their stories support the need for a systems approach to professional well-being as recommended by the National Academy of Medicine.[1]

ASSESSMENT AND MEASUREMENT TOOLS

One of the recommendations of the National Academy of Medicine report is that we use validated measurement tools to assess the current state of burnout, professional well-being, and factors related to stress and well-being.[1] Measurement can occur at the individual level as well as the unit and organizational level. Measurement plans can range from self-assessment that provides the individual nurse with confidential, evidence-based feedback and self-help guidance to a broader (unit or organization-wide) assessment of culture.[25,26] Regardless of the chosen assessment model, the goal is to identify important opportunities for intervention.

Table 1 includes examples of assessments tools that could be used with critical care nurses. In addition to including measures that tap into positive psychology constructs (meaning and joy, happiness, self-compassion, resilience, and well-being), measures of anxiety, depression, trauma, alcohol use, and health care provider distress are also included due to their direct relationship with one's capacity to experience joy and to connect with others. Finally, an assessment of organizational sources of support and the effectiveness of those resources is included in the table for a team or organization-wide evaluation that can be used to address perceived weaknesses in established support systems or to assess improvements due to support interventions, such as the implementation of peer support programs.

INTERVENTIONS

There are many studies of interventions to promote various aspects of well-being. These studies evaluate the effectiveness of clinical interventions designed for individuals with

Table 1
Measurement tools

Measure	Construct	# Items
Meaning and Joy in Work Questionnaire (MJWQ)[34]	Three subscales include value/ connections, meaningful work, and caring	17
Subjective Happiness Scale (SHS)[35]	Perceived happiness	4
Self-Compassion Scale-Short Form (SCS-SF)[36]	Overall score & 6 subscores: self-kindness; self-judgement, common humanity; isolation; mindfulness; overidentification	12
Brief Resilience Scale (BRS)[25,37]	Ability to bounce back or recover from stress	6
Nurse Well-being Index (WBI)[38]	Burnout, fatigue, low mental/physical quality of life, depression, anxiety/ stress, satisfaction with work life integration; meaning in work	9
Primary Care PTSD Screen (PC-PTSD)[25,39]	Posttraumatic stress disorder (PTSD) symptoms	4
Patient Health Questionnaire-2 (PHQ-2)[25,40,41]	Depression	2
Generalized Anxiety Disorder-7 (GAD-7)[25,31,42]	Generalized worry anxiety	7
Measure of Moral Distress for Healthcare Professionals (MMD-HP)[43]	Four factors: futile care, poor teamwork, deceptive communication, ethical misconduct	27
Alcohol Use Disorders Identification Test (AUDIT)[44]	Frequency and amount of consumption	10
Medically Induced Trauma Support Services (MTSS) Staff Support Assessment Tool[26]	Environmental assessment of support resources and their effectiveness (including peer support)	67

mental health concerns to organizational interventions designed to mitigate burnout among health professionals. Jarden and colleagues[27] studied the experience of New Zealand critical care nurses with factors that strengthened nurse well-being. Their findings include "strengtheners" at the individual or "Me" level, the unit or "We" level, and the organizational of "Us"level.[27(p17)] Their recommendations align with the recommendations of critical care nurses described earlier, the American Association of Critical Care Nurses (AACN) healthy work environment framework,[28] the IHI Joy in Work framework,[8] and the National Academy of Medicine recommendations for a systems approach to professional well-being.[1] There are many similarities in these evidence-based recommendations indicating consensus on the multipronged strategy required to promote professional well-being. They are summarized in **Table 2**.

Me—Interventions for Individual Nurses

At the individual level, nurses and their health care colleagues can engage in self-care strategies that will enhance their resilience and well-being and decrease the risk of

Table 2
Recommendations to strengthen clinician well-being

A Narrative Analysis of Nurses' Experiences with Meaning and Joy in Nursing Practice[16]	Strengthening Workplace Well-Being[27]	AACN Standards for Establishing and Sustaining Healthy Work Environments[28]	IHI Joy in Work Framework[8]	Taking Action Against Clinician Burnout: a Systems Approach to Professional Well-Being[1]
Individual-level Interventions				
Self-care practices	Self-care practices		Cultivating own wellness and resilience (self-care)	Mindfulness, stress management, small-group discussions
Schedule management	Schedule management, "Simplifying life," work-life balance			
Spiritual practices	Spiritual practices			
Exercise	Exercise, yoga			Exercise
Engage in professional governance councils and improvement work		Engage in collaborative decision-making processes, participate in established forums	Identify opportunities to improve, be part of the solution, speak up	Human-centered co-design, participatory decision-making, clinician engagement, autonomy
Pursue development opportunities		Identify learning needs and seek opportunities to improve communication, collaboration, and clinical competence	Commitment to doing their best and continuous improvement	Resiliency training
Team and Leader-level Interventions				

Get to know each nurse as a person. Ask why they chose nursing, what they find meaningful, and what brings them joy.		Invite and hear all perspectives	Ask "what matters to you?" to understand meaning and purpose for each person	Resonant and authentic leadership, alignment of values and behaviors
Listen and help nurses to make the connection between their practice and their sense of purpose, values, and identity.		Leaders translate the vision of a healthy work environment	"Daily work is connected to what called individuals to practice, line of sight to organization mission and goals" (pp 17–18)	Eliminate low-value work and enhance meaning and purpose of work
Create opportunities for sharing stories of meaning and joy. Leaders share their experiences.		Leaders generate enthusiasm and role model skilled communication, meaningful recognition, and authentic leadership		Resonant and authentic leadership
Co-create a practice environment that values and supports both the science and the art of nursing.	Continuing education and development opportunities			
Co-design practices to increase the time nurses spend with patients and families to establish therapeutic relationships and individualize care.	"Job crafting" (p 18)	Leaders design systems to implement and sustain healthy work environments	Participative management and shared governance encourage voice and empower clinicians to drive change. Leaders create space to listen, understand, and involve	Human-centered work system redesign with clinicians. Optimize workload and task distribution

(continued on next page)

Table 2
(continued)

A Narrative Analysis of Nurses' Experiences with Meaning and Joy in Nursing Practice[16]	Strengthening Workplace Well-Being[27]	AACN Standards for Establishing and Sustaining Healthy Work Environments[28]	IHI Joy in Work Framework[8]	Taking Action Against Clinician Burnout: a Systems Approach to Professional Well-Being[1]
Co-create the conditions for nurses to form meaningful connections with one another and members of the interprofessional team.	Promotion of teamwork, mutual support, collaboration, effective communication	RN and MD leaders model and foster true collaboration; every team member embraces true collaboration	Social cohesion through productive teams, shared understanding, and trusting relationships	Facilitate interprofessional teamwork, collaboration, communication, and professionalism
Establish processes for peer and patient/family recognition and appreciation. Consistently celebrate meaningful contributions.	Regular encouragement and appreciation	Team members recognize one another in a meaningful way for their contributions	Regular meaningful recognition of colleagues' contribution to purpose and celebration of outcomes	Meaningful recognition, opportunities to hear from patients and families
Encourage and reward creativity, innovation, professional autonomy, and risk-taking.			Psychological safety, respectful climate, can take risks, speak up, admit mistakes, seek feedback Allow for choice and flexibility in daily lives and work	Psychological safety, atmosphere of learning, co-creation of solutions

Organization-level Interventions

Safe staffing levels	Appropriate staffing including policies, decision-making processes, evaluation, and improvement		Schedule and staffing changes, reductions in workload intensity
Fair compensation	Performance appraisals include HWE behavioral expectations	Fair and equitable systems	Rewards and compensation systems support well-being
Training resources	Education programs and coaching to improve communication skills		CREW training to promote civility, healthy relationships, and trust
Psychological support structures. Zero tolerance for bullying	Formal structures that ensure respectful information sharing. Zero-tolerance for disrespectful behavior and abuse	"Equitable environment, free from harm, just culture that is, safe and respectful, support for the second victim"	Social support, discussion groups, alignment of values, and behaviors
Wellness programs (physical and psychological health)		Physical and psychological safety is a precondition for joy in work. Senior leader champion, set the vision and model the way, leaders at all levels commit to promoting joy in work and well-being (holistic approach)	Infrastructure for enhancing well-being with executive leader (Chief Wellness Officer). Efforts coordinated with patient and employee safety programs

(continued on next page)

Table 2
(continued)

A Narrative Analysis of Nurses' Experiences with Meaning and Joy in Nursing Practice[16]	Strengthening Workplace Well-Being[27]	AACN Standards for Establishing and Sustaining Healthy Work Environments[28]	IHI Joy in Work Framework[8]	Taking Action Against Clinician Burnout: a Systems Approach to Professional Well-Being[1]
	Recognition programs for individuals and groups	Comprehensive system for meaningful recognition of all team members	Comprehensive, nontraditional approach to meaningful recognition and appreciation	Meaningful recognition programs Participation in Magnet Recognition Program, Pathway to Excellence Program, Joy in Medicine Recognition Program
		Systematic evaluation and design of staffing, support services, and technology use to increase the efficiency of work and to match patient needs and nursing care	Use improvement science to identify, test, and implement improvements	Human-centered work system redesign. Improve distribution of tasks, participatory decision-making, evaluate, and improve use of technology to reduce work burden
		Regularly measure progress toward HWE using validated tools, evaluate impact, take action to improve	Measurement systems enable regular feedback about system performance to facilitate improvement	Establish assessment strategies using validated instruments with regular review of data and action steps
		Authentic leadership	"High-Impact Leadership" behaviors	Accessible authentic and resonant leaders Leadership engagement at all levels and across all disciplines to create the conditions for clinician well-being

| Leadership development programs | Leadership development programs to support HWE, including formal mentoring | Facilitation of HWE by providing time and financial and human resources | Senior leaders create the culture, ensure system effectiveness, commit to improvement, and celebrate outcomes | Adoption of evidence-based healthy work environment strategies |

burnout. These include strategies to promote physical health as well as psychological well-being. Physical exercise, yoga, a healthy diet, and sleep are some of the recommended wellness-promotion activities. Mindfulness, gratitude practice, and spiritual practices along with schedule management have been found to enhance well-being and increase resilience.[29–31] Studies indicate that nurses and their colleagues are aware of these self-care strategies and many are working to incorporate these into their lives and practice to promote their own health and well-being and prevent illness and burnout.[8,27] Specific coping skills that improve resilience include self-awareness and reflection using narrative techniques, inspirational goal-setting, problem-solving, emotion regulation techniques, boundary setting, communication skills with highly distressed individuals, and the development of positive social support networks.[25]

We—Team-Based Interventions

At the team level, evidence-based recommendations for leaders and health care team members are consistent with the 6 elements of the AACN healthy work environment standards.[28] Authentic leadership is an essential driver of practice environment improvement and sustainability. Nurse leaders set the stage for adoption and enculturation of healthy relationships with skilled communication, true collaboration, and decision-making. They assure that resources, including staffing, support the ability of nurses and teams to provide care in a meaningful way. They also provide meaningful recognition and assure that it is a core component of the team culture. They engage and empower nurses and interprofessional colleagues in co-creating and co-designing care delivery to align with values and assure meaningful work. The recommendations are consistent from the voices of nurses in qualitative studies, to professional organization frameworks, to the National Academy of Medicine call to action. There is substantial evidence-based guidance for teams and leaders to engage in action planning and implementation to create the practice environments that will bring them meaning and joy and promote their well-being. Team-based and hospital-wide interventions designed to militate against the chronic stress and trauma of critical care work, such as skilled peer support programs that are activated after an adverse patient event, have been of particular interest to the Joint Commission.[32,33]

Us—Organizational Level Interventions

There is substantial agreement that interventions at the individual and the local team level are insufficient to produce the effects on clinician well-being that are required. Entire organizations and the health care system must engage in transformational change to reverse the growing epidemic of clinician burnout and disengagement. The systems approach outlined by the National Academy of Medicine provides a roadmap for a collaborative, multilevel plan to redesign the health care system to assure that it is human-centered with high-quality care for patients and flourishing health care professionals.

SUMMARY

Healthy nurses are essential for improved population health, better patient care experiences, and cost reduction in our health care system.[1] Meaning and joy in nursing practice are contributors to professional well-being and are part of the solution for achieving the quadruple aim. Emerging models for addressing nursing well-being are consistent with the larger psychological literature. Validated assessment approaches, evidence-based interventions and support resources, and organizational commitment are key features of a successful approach for achieving the quadruple aim.

DISCLOSURE

The authors have nothing to disclose.

REFERENCES

1. National Academies of Sciences, Engineering, and Medicine. Taking action against clinician burnout: a systems approach to professional well-being. Washington, DC: The National Academies Press; 2019.
2. Berwick DM, Nolan TW, Whittington J. The triple aim: care, health, and cost. HealthAff 2008;27(3):759–69.
3. Sikka R, Morath JM, Leape L. The Quadruple Aim: care, health, cost and meaning in work. BMJQualSaf 2015;24(10):608–10.
4. Seligman MEP. Flourish: a visionary new understanding of happiness and well-being. New York: Atria Paperback; 2013.
5. Achor S. The happiness advantage: how a positive brain fuels success in work and life. New York: Currency; 2018.
6. Moss J, Achor S. Unlocking happiness at work: how a Data-Driven happiness strategy fuels purpose, passion and performance. London: Kogan Page; 2016.
7. Gilbert D, Morse G. The science behind the smile. Harvard Business Review 2012. Available at: https://hbr.org/2012/01/the-science-behind-the-smile?ab=hbra-257. Accessed November 12, 2019.
8. Perlo J, Balik B, Swenson S, et al. IHI framework for improving joy in work. IHI white paper. Cambridge (MA): Institute for Healthcare Improvement; 2017.
9. Csikszentmihalyi M. Flow: the psychology of optimal experience. New York: Harper Row; 2009.
10. Health care workforce special report: the state of engagement." press Ganey. Available at: www.pressganey.com/resources/white-papers/health-care-workforce-special-report-the-state-of-engagement. Accessed December 1, 2019.
11. Bargagliotti LA. Work engagement in nursing: a concept analysis. J AdvNurs 2011;68(6):1414–28.
12. Rivera RR, Fitzpatrick JJ, Boyle SM. Closing the RN engagement Gap. J Nurs Adm 2011;41(6):265–72.
13. Dempsey C, Reilly BA. Nurse engagement: what are the contributing factors for success? Online J IssuesNurs 2016;21:1. Accessed November 12, 2019.
14. Koloroutis M, Abelson D. Advancing relationship-based cultures. Minneapolis (MN): Creative health care management; 2018.
15. Santos A, Castanheira F, Chambel MJ, et al. Relational job characteristics and well-being: a study among Portuguese and Brazilian hospital nurses. Stress Health 2016;33(4):415–25.
16. Galuska L, Hahn J, Polifroni EC, et al. A narrative analysis of nurses' experiences with meaning and joy in nursing practice. NursAdm Q 2018;42(2):154–63.
17. Benzo RP, Kirsch JL, Nelson C. Compassion, mindfulness, and the happiness of healthcare workers. Explore (NY) 2017;13(3):201–6.
18. Durkin M, Beaumont E, Martin CJH, et al. A pilot study exploring the relationship between self-compassion, self-judgement, self-kindness, compassion, professional quality of life and wellbeing among UK community nurses. Nurse Educ Today 2016;46:109–14.

19. Andrews H, Tierney S, Seers K. Needing permission: the experience of self-care and self-compassion in nursing: a constructivist grounded theory study. Int J Nurs Stud 2020;101:103436.

20. Quinn R, Thakor AV. Creating a purpose-Driven organization. Harvard Business Review 2018. Available at: https://hbr.org/2018/07/creating-a-purpose-driven-organization?autocomplete=true. Accessed November 12, 2019.

21. Tong L. Relationship between meaningful work and job performance in nurses. Int J NursPract 2018;24(2). https://doi.org/10.1111/ijn.12620.

22. Ziedelis A. Perceived calling and work engagement among nurses. West J Nurs Res 2018;41(6):816–33.

23. Fontaine DK, Haizlip J, Lavandero R. No time to be nice in the intensive care unit. Am J CritCare 2018;27(2):153–6.

24. Shanafelt TD, West CP, Sloan JA, et al. Career fit and burnout among academic faculty. Arch Intern Med 2009;169(10):990.

25. Bursch B, Emerson ND, Arevian AC, et al. Feasibility of online mental wellness self-assessment and feedback for pediatric and neonatal critical care nurses. J PediatrNurs 2018;43:62–8.

26. Download the toolkit. MITSS. Available at: http://mitss.org/download-the-toolkit. Accessed November 11, 2019.

27. Jarden RJ, Sandham M, Siegert RJ, et al. Strengthening workplace well-being: perceptions of intensive care nurses. NursCritCare 2018;24(1):15–23.

28. AACN Standards for Establishing and Maintaining Healthy Work Environments. A journey to excellence, 2nd edition 2015. Available at: www.aacn.org/nursing-excellence/standards/aacn-standards-for-establishing-and-sustaining-healthy-work-environments. Accessed December 17, 2019.

29. Benzo RP, Anderson PM, Bronars C, et al. Mindfulness for healthcare providers: the role of non-reactivity in reducing stress. Explore (NY) 2018;14(6):453–6.

30. Berkland BE, Werneburg BL, Jenkins SM, et al. A worksite wellness intervention: improving happiness, life satisfaction, and gratitude in health care workers. Mayo ClinProcInnovQualOutcomes 2017;1(3):203–10.

31. Watanabe N, Furukawa TA, Horikoshi M, et al. A mindfulness-based stress management program and treatment with omega-3 fatty acids to maintain a healthy mental state in hospital nurses (Happy Nurse Project): study protocol for a randomized controlled trial. Trials 2015;16(1). https://doi.org/10.1186/s13063-015-0554-z.

32. Quick safety issue 39. The Joint Commission. Available at: https://www.jointcommission.org/resources/news-and-multimedia/newsletters/newsletters/quick-safety/quick-safety-issue-39-supporting-second-victims/. Accessed December 17, 2019.

33. Pratt S, Kenney L, Scott SD, et al. How to develop a second victim support program: a toolkit for health care organizations. JtComm J QualPatientSaf 2012;38(5):235–40.

34. Rutledge DN, Wickman M, Winokur EJ. Instrument validation: hospital nurse perceptions of meaning and joy in work. J Nurs Meas 2018;26(3):579–88.

35. Lyubomirsky S, Lepper HS. A measure of subjective happiness: preliminary reliability and construct validation. Soc Indic Res 1999;46(2):137–55.

36. Raes F, Pommier E, Neff KD, et al. Construction and factorial validation of a short form of the Self-Compassion Scale. ClinPsycholPsychother 2010;18(3):250–5.

37. Smith BW, Dalen J, Wiggins K, et al. The brief resilience scale: assessing the ability to bounce back. Int J Behav Med 2008;15(3):194–200.

38. Dyrbye LN, Johnson PO, Johnson LM, et al. Efficacy of the well-being index to identify distress and well-being in U.S. Nurses. Nurs Res 2018;67(6):447–55.

39. Prins A, Ouimette P, Kimerling R, et al. The primary care PTSD screen (PC-PTSD): development and operating characteristics. Primary Care Psychiatry 2004;9(1):9–14.

40. Kroenke K, Spitzer RL, Williams JBW. The patient health Questionnaire-2. Med Care 2003;41(11):1284–92.

41. Tsaras K, Papathanasiou I, Vus V, et al. Predicting factors of depression and anxiety in mental health nurses: a quantitative cross-sectional study. Med Arch 2018; 72(1):62.

42. Spitzer RL, Kroenke K, Williams JBW, et al. A brief measure for assessing generalized anxiety disorder. Arch Intern Med 2006;166(10):1092.

43. Epstein EG, Whitehead PB, Prompahakul C, et al. Enhancingunderstanding of moral distress: the measure of moral distress for health care professionals. AJOBEmpirBioeth 2019;10(2):113–24.

44. Leung SF, Arthur D. The alcohol use disorders identification test (AUDIT): validation of an instrument for enhancing nursing practice in Hong Kong. Int J Nurs Stud 2000;37(1):57–64.

Replenish at Work

An Integrative Program to Decrease Stress and Promote a Culture of Wellness in the Intensive Care Unit

Catherine Alvarez, MA, BS, RN, CNML, HNB-BC, PCCN*

KEYWORDS

• Burnout • Self-care • Mindfulness • Wellness program • Critical care

KEY POINTS

- Supporting intensive care unit (ICU) staff through the promotion of self-care and mindfulness programs is successful in improving stress and burnout and in promoting resilience.
- Addressing barriers to engaging in self-care practices and identifying unit-specific needs are crucial to creating successful wellness programs.
- Providing wellness interventions, such as microrestorative practices, has the potential to alleviate the immediate stress generated from patient care and provide a moment of peace.
- Leadership and organizational support are vital in identifying the need for and promoting wellness programs for staff.

INTRODUCTION

Health care workers face numerous stressors in the workday. Specifically, intensive care unit (ICU) nurses are exposed to unique demands, including excessive workloads, managing end-of-life concerns and prolonged care, and moral distress related to ethical issues.[1–3] With increasing demands on time, resources, and energy, it is not surprising that ICU nurses report some of the highest rates of stress and burnout. The estimated rate of burnout among ICU nurses is between 25% and 80%,[4] and these high levels of burnout have a significant negative impact on employee health and well-being.

Burnout is a state of mental, physical, and emotional exhaustion caused by prolonged exposure to stress in the workplace and is characterized by overwhelming exhaustion, detachment from work, and a lack of sense of personal accomplishment.[5] Burnout affects all aspects of health and can lead to anxiety and depression,

Yale New Haven Hospital, New Haven, CT, USA
* 300 George Street, Cube 142, New Haven, CT 06511.
E-mail address: catherine.alvarez@ynhh.org

Crit Care Nurs Clin N Am 32 (2020) 369–381
https://doi.org/10.1016/j.cnc.2020.05.001
0899-5885/20/Published by Elsevier Inc.

substance abuse, and suicidal ideations.[6] Furthermore, caregiver burnout can have an impact on organizations through decreased productivity, increased risk of workplace accidents, decreased staff engagement, absenteeism, intent to leave practice, and turnover.[1,7,8] Nurse absenteeism and turnover caused by stress can lead to inadequate staffing and can put patient safety in jeopardy. The purpose of the current pilot study is to assess the feasibility of a Replenish at Work program to reduce the impact of a stressful environment on Cardiothoracic ICU (CTICU) personnel.

BACKGROUND

In 2005, the American Association for Critical-Care Nurses (AACN) released the *AACN Standards for Establishing and Sustaining Healthy Work Environments: A Journey to Excellence*.[9] Recognizing that unhealthy work environments contribute to stress, conflict, medical errors, and inefficiencies in care delivery, the document called attention to the need to foster healthy work environments to combat stress, improve recruitment and retention, and ensure patient safety and quality outcomes. Each standard is considered essential and fundamental to promoting healthy work environments (**Box 1**). In 2016, the AACN released a second edition of the document, focusing on the 6 essential standards but also providing a blueprint of critical elements needed for organizations and leaders to use to implement specific practices.[10]

A recent evaluation of the critical care nurse work environments was completed in 2018.[11] Results of the study conducted on 8080 (AACN) members revealed that work environments for critical care nurses have improved in many of the 6 essential domains. Opportunities to enhance the critical care work environment, however, remain in relation to job satisfaction, intent to leave, and physical and mental well-being of the critical care nurse.[11] The percentage of ICU nurses who reported experiencing moral distress in the 2018 survey (10.6%) increased from 2013 (9.4%). Moral distress is an emotional state that arises when a nurse feels the actions needed for patients differ from what is ethically correct. High levels of moral distress have been associated with decreased job satisfaction and can contribute further to symptoms of burnout.[11]

Although stress and burnout have been well documented and studied among ICU nurses, studies testing interventions to address the problem are scarce. Most studies evaluate the effects of individual-focused strategies and provide little information to indicate efficacy.[12] Other studies suggest that fostering stress management through self-care training and mindfulness interventions isare beneficial.[6] Self-care is defined

---

Box 1
American Association for Critical-Care Nurses standards for establishing and sustaining healthy work environments

1. Skilled communication

2. True collaboration

3. Effective decision making

4. Meaningful recognition

5. Appropriate staffing

6. Authentic leadership

Data from American Association of Critical-Care Nurses. AACN standards for establishing and sustaining healthy work environments: a journey to excellence. 2nd ed. Aliso Viejo, CA: American Association of Critical-Care Nurses; 2016.

as the "practice of engaging in health-related activities and using health-promoting behaviors to adopt a healthier lifestyle and enhance wellness."[13] A core value of holistic nursing is a commitment to self-care and self-reflection in order to provide healing for others.[14] Using self-reflection, nurses learn how to pause, reflect on their needs, and practice centering and stress-reduction techniques. When nurses engage in self-care practices, they not only function and manage stress better but also are able to deliver high-quality care.[15] Because nurses have been trained to prioritize patient needs before their own, however, it is questionable whether nurses will practice self-care if they are not trained or required to do so. Additionally, research has shown many nurses avoid taking care of their own physical or mental needs for fear of stigma or retaliatory responses.[16,17] Furthermore, nursing knowledge regarding self-care often is lacking. The absence of self-care practices can increase stress levels and further contribute to burnout as well as having a negative impact on patient outcomes.[18,19] Therefore, it is imperative to make the importance of self-care visible and more valued in practice through wellness programs. Leadership and organizational support are vital to initiating this process.

Studies investigating wellness programs and practices that support psychological and spiritual well-being have been shown to result in greater resilience.[20–22] Specifically, researchers have found self-care practices consisting of instructor-led mindfulness and/or mindfulness-based stress reduction practices are effective in managing stress and burnout and promoting resilience.[23] Mindfulness is "paying attention, in a particular way: on purpose, in the present moment, and non-judgmentally."[24] The goals of mindfulness are to improve self-awareness, active listening, presence, and compassion.[25] Mindfulness interventions can be associated with reductions in stress, anxiety, and depression in addition to reducing burnout.[26,27] Specifically, in the ICU setting, Steinberg and colleagues[28] (2017) found that an 8-week workplace mindfulness intervention, consisting of gentle yoga movements, meditation, and music, increased work satisfaction and engagement scores among surgical ICU nurses. Additionally, a simple 5-minute mindfulness intervention provided to pediatric ICU nurses before the start of a shift for 30 days reduced nurse stress.[29] Although the immediate effect of these interventions on individual stress and resiliency is clear, the long-term benefits of these programs remain unknown.

Organizational support is needed to target interventions aimed at reducing burnout on an individual level. Press Ganey Associates (2018)[30] emphasized that the success of interventions is determined by how leadership addresses the problem of burnout. If organizations believe burnout is strictly an individual problem and do not take accountability for the processes that produce stress and burnout, success at creating healthy work environments and promoting resilience will fail. Wellness interventions aimed at both the individual and organization levels, therefore, are imperative to support the ongoing demands of the nurse.

Studies on evidence-based strategies to support organization interventions for nurses need further development. A systematic review of interventions to prevent and reduce physician burnout confirmed the need for both individual-focused (ie, personal stress reduction and resilience training) and organizational strategies.[7] From an organizational standpoint thus far, successful interventions focusing on the reduction of clerical work,[31] modifying workplaces via improvements in workflow and communication, and using quality-improvement projects to specifically target clinician concerns have resulted in lower levels of burnout for clinicians.[32] In nursing practice, particularly in ICUs, organizational approaches should focus on improving work conditions, such as appropriate staffing and resources to buffer high workloads[33] and improving meaningful recognition from leadership.[34]

ORGANIZATION STRATEGIES TO REDUCE BURNOUT

Two organizations, Stanford Medicine and the Mayo Clinic, have been pioneers in utilizing both individual and organizational support to improve health care well-being. The Stanford Model for Professional Fulfillment and Worksite Wellness (**Fig. 1**) cites 3 domains that organizations needed to achieve well-being for health care professionals.[35] The 3 domains are inclusive and represent the importance of organizations creating an environment that values and supports self-care and self-compassion; improving workplace systems, processes, and practices to promote quality care and work-life balance; and encouraging behaviors that contribute to personal, physical, spiritual, and emotional well-being.

In addition to the Stanford Model, the Mayo Clinic has successfully implemented 9 organizational strategies to promote executive leadership and physician well-being and reduce burnout[36] (**Box 2**). Incorporating these 9 organizational strategies has resulted in a reduction of burnout below national average, despite having to improve efficiencies, decrease costs, and increase productivity,[37] and further supports the research that healthier work environments are associated with lower levels of burnout.[34]

PROGRAM DEVELOPMENT

Leadership support is crucial in promoting a healthy work environment and creating interventions to support and promote resiliency.[37] The vice president (VP) of nursing for the heart and vascular and transplantation department in a large academic Magnet® organization identified a critical need among CTICU staff. During leader rounds and open forums with staff and the local management team, an increase in stress, turnover, and low morale was identified. The CTICU is an 18-bed unit that provides care for critically ill patients who have undergone cardiothoracic surgeries. Patient care in this unit was getting increasingly complex. Staffing the unit to meet the multifaceted patient needs, however, was becoming a challenge.

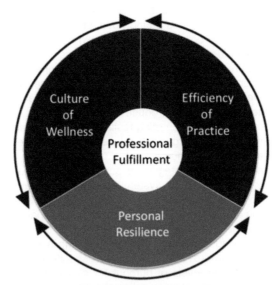

Fig. 1. Stanford Model for Professional Fulfillment in Health Care Professionals. (© 2016 The Board of Trustees of the Leland Stanford Junior University. All rights reserved. Used with permission.)

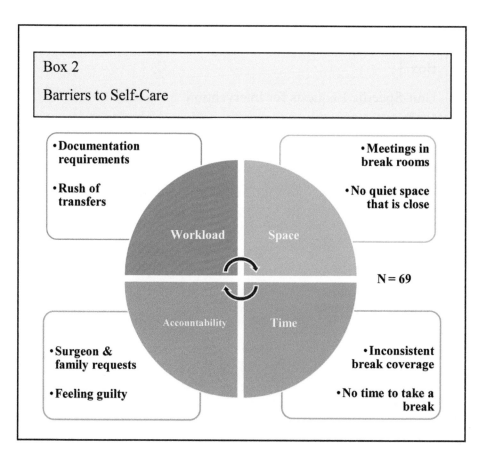

Box 2

Barriers to Self-Care

- **Documentation requirements**
- **Rush of transfers**

Workload

Space

- **Meetings in break rooms**
- **No quiet space that is close**

N = 69

Accountability

Time

- **Surgeon & family requests**
- **Feeling guilty**

- **Inconsistent break coverage**
- **No time to take a break**

The VP of nursing proposed using benefactor donor funds to create a wellness and resiliency program targeting the CTICU staff. Two holistic nurses experienced in developing curricula focusing on resiliency were recruited to design and implement a mindfulness-based intervention that they called Replenish at Work. One nurse was a full-time staff member at the organization and the other was an independent contractor. The VP and patient services manager (PSM) of the unit offered unit-specific data to the facilitators, and collaboration began regarding budget and program design and schedule. To maximize the organization's return on investment and determine targeted wellness interventions for the unit, the facilitators conducted a needs assessment.

A total of 69 staff members, including nurses, patient care associates, and business associates (75% of staff), representing all shifts participated in the needs assessment. Results demonstrated current barriers to self-care practices as well as unit-specific needs to promote self-care; 75% of staff self-reported they did not have a practice in place to care for themselves during the shift, whereas the other 25% reported self-care practices of bathroom use, food, and drink. These data are consistent with literature demonstrating the lack of self-care practices among nurses and its consequential impact on burnout.[18]

Barriers to self-care reported from the CTICU staff were collated and themed into 4 categories: workload, space, time, and accountability (**Box 3**). The facilitators reported

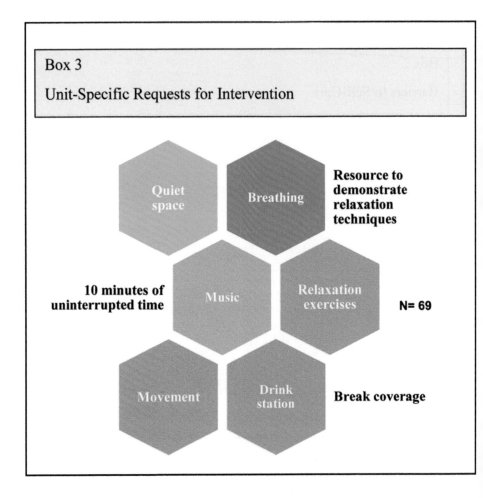

Box 3

Unit-Specific Requests for Intervention

Quiet space

Breathing

Resource to demonstrate relaxation techniques

10 minutes of uninterrupted time

Music

Relaxation exercises

N= 69

Movement

Drink station

Break coverage

these results and unit-specific requests (**Box 4**) to the VP of nursing and PSM to gain support and further collaborate on the intervention and preferred length of delivery. Staff request for personnel coverage during the intervention was addressed with the leadership team. After reviewing the literature supporting the need for staff coverage during on-site interventions,[28] administration agreed to have a per diem nurse provide additional coverage.

The purpose of the current pilot study was to assess the feasibility of a Replenish at Work program to reduce the impact of a stressful environment on CTICU personnel. The program was grounded in Jean Watson's Theory of Human Caring and Clinical Caritas Processes. The Theory of Human Caring emphasizes the need for caring for self as imperative to holistically and authentically caring for patients.[15] Additionally, Watson's Clinical Caritas Processes describe the importance of being authentically present, supporting both positive and negative feelings, and creating healing environments for patients.[38] Nurses' care for self and care for others are interdependent. Without love and respect for self, they are unlikely to be able to care for others with compassion and understanding. It was hypothesized that developing

---

Box 4
Strategies to promote leadership and physician well-being and reduce burnout

1. Acknowledge and assess the problem

2. Harness the power of leadership

3. Develop and implement targeted work unit interventions

4. Cultivate community at work

5. Use rewards and incentives wisely

6. Align values and strengthen the culture

7. Promote flexibility and work-life integration

8. Provide resources to promote resilience and self-care strategies

9. Facilitate and fund organizational science

Data from Shanafelt TD, Noseworthy JH. Executive leadership and physician well-being. Mayo Clin Proc. 2017;92(1):129–46.

---

self-awareness and self-care practices through a brief mindfulness intervention would improve stress levels and promote resiliency among CTICU staff.

The Replenish at Work curriculum was informed by the works of Sitzman and Watson,[39] Neff and Germer,[40] and Siegel.[41] A combination of didactic teaching, facilitator-led group discussion, and mindfulness practices designed to cultivate self-care through mindful awareness and self-compassion aimed at strengthening focused attention and presence were used. The curriculum included an overarching lesson on the importance of self-care and self-reflection, followed by mindfulness exercises incorporating breath awareness and mindful movements, called microrestorative practices (**Box 5**). These short practices are intentional breaks that combine stillness, breath awareness, and movement to gain clarity, connection, and compassion to bring peace amidst chaos. Managing stress also was discussed briefly, including

---

Box 5
Replenish at Work content outline

30-minute session
 Purpose: to understand the importance of self-care and learn the basics of mindfulness
 practice
 Learning outcomes
 • Examine the cause and effect of stress
 • Identify barriers to self-care and personal self-care needs
 • Explore strategies to create a healthier work environment
 • Discuss the importance of mindfulness practices
 Participants learned the basics of mindfulness, self-awareness, and self-compassion as tools
 for self-care. Breath work and mindful movement were introduced to relieve tension and
 cultivate positive states of mind.

10-minute session
 Purpose: to expand self-care and mindfulness practice through experiential microrestorative
 movements
 Learning outcomes
 • Recognize stress signals in the mind and body
 • Engage in self-management techniques
 Participants utilized breathe awareness and movement to perform microrestorative practices
 relevant to individual needs

developing intentional awareness of self-care needs and practicing gratitude. Light music, fruit-infused water to hydrate, and essential oil–infused lotion were provided to promote a restorative environment conducive of a mindful break and meet unit requests identified in the needs assessment (see **Box 4**).

REPLENISH AT WORK PROGRAM

The Replenish at Work program was conducted in a small office space on site in the CTICU over the course of 4 weeks. Timing of the intervention was designed to meet staff member needs across all shifts, including weekends and nights. This ensured the intervention was part of the work shift and not an additional burden for staff. At the request of the VP and PSM, all staff members (registered nurses, patient care associates, and business associates) were included in the intervention if they were currently working in the CTICU setting. No exclusion criteria were specified, and participation was voluntary. A sign-in log identified the number of participants.

The facilitators and per diem nurse were scheduled in 3-hour intervals 5 times a week to promote staff attendance in the 30-minute sessions. Education was provided by 2 trained holistic nurses and mindfulness experts and delivered in a ratio of 1 instructor to 2:3 CTICU staff members. This delivery method was chosen to foster a sense of community and social support among staff. Additionally, more intimate and individual training is more effective in promoting resilience than classroom-based delivery methods.[42] The initial intervention consisted of a 30-minute introduction, followed by a combination of self-care and mindfulness practices. After all participants received the 30-minute intervention, a 10-minute follow-up session was conducted to heighten awareness in the applicability of the microrestorative practices. These brief interventions were adapted to meet the ongoing time constraints identified by CTICU team members and were intended to become integrated in the workplace. It was suggested that participants attend at least one 10-minute experiential follow-up session. An anonymous postintervention survey was conducted 2 weeks after the last 10-minute session to assess participant feedback and feasibility of the program.

PROGRAM OUTCOMES

The intervention team was able to provide initial 30-minute sessions to 93% (n = 86) of CTICU staff members over the course of 2 weeks. During the next 2 weeks, each participant received at least one 10-minute session. Most staff members participated in at least two 10-minute sessions, whereas a few received three to five 10-minute interventions (**Fig. 2**). The overall cost for the Replenish at Work program was $10,000. This cost included 60 hours of instructional time for the independent contractor as well as 60 per diem staff nurse hours. The cost of the other facilitator was absorbed in her full-time hours.

A total of 56 staff members (60%) completed the postintervention survey. Data collected revealed anecdotal evidence of the benefit of the program. When asked about the intervention, 62% of staff members responded positively, referring to the intervention as refreshing, helpful, enlightening, and relevant to practice. One participant noted, "I think the sessions were very helpful. Even though 10 minutes can seem like a long time if you have a lot of tasks at hand, it was helpful to step away from the stressful environment and it decreased my stress level for the rest of the shift." Another stated, "I thought that it was helpful. I would have to say the most beneficial part was just reminding me to be aware of myself. I think that the interventions taught are easy to practice and I will incorporate them in my routine." All 100% of staff were grateful someone could relieve them while participating in the intervention. However, 35% still

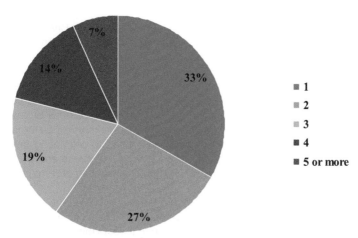

Fig. 2. Graphical representation of 10-minute session attendance.

felt compelled to return to their job as soon as possible and 3% did not think the intervention was relevant to the unit's needs. Music, fruit-infused water, and ease of the microrestorative movements were reported as beneficial.

Among respondents, 65% of individuals stated the program was effective in improving their ability to better manage their job and take care of patients after focusing on their self-care needs. Despite the unit location, there was a desire for a more private and quieter place to conduct the intervention. Increasing the frequency of intervention, continuing to provide personnel coverage for the intervention as well as routine break time, and incorporating more music also were cited as suggestions for improvement.

Among respondents, 93% affirmed the Replenish at Work program should be shared across all departments and found the intervention helpful in promoting self-care practices and improving stress. Participants cited the potential long-term benefits of an intervention in lessening stress to promote better health, patient care results, and retention of nurses. The support of leadership was critical to the success of this program. Many respondents noted the success and sustainability of such a program would be dependent on leadership and organizational support. One participant reiterated this by stating, "It felt good to know that someone cares about us and recognizes that without change, stress and burnout will continue."

An institutional employee engagement survey conducted 2 months after the 4-week intervention showed a 14.3% improvement compared with the previous year. Although engagement was not a direct measurement tool in this study, results are promising and may warrant future investigation on the impact of self-care and mindfulness practices with regard to staff engagement.

Limitations of the study include the lack of a control group, small sample size, and that all participants were employed in a single organization. Other limitations include the self-reported nature of the program, which could be subject to respondent bias. Additionally, the Replenish at Work program was not measured longitudinally over time. In order to provide self-care and resiliency programs such as this, staffing needs to be enhanced representing costs organizations need to consider.

DISCUSSION

Nurses working in high-risk and acute care areas, such as the ICU, are at increased risk for stress and burnout. The high percentage of voluntary participants indicates a strong interest among ICU nurses in participating in self-care programs. Brief microrestorative practices are effective in gaining clarity, connection, and compassion and in bringing peace amidst the chaos. Program feedback highlighted an improvement in self-reported stress levels and self-care practices. In addition, participants reported the ability to provide better care for their patients after a brief pause to care for themselves.

Addressing barriers to engaging in self-care practices and identifying unit-specific needs are crucial to creating wellness programs. These can be done by assessing individual levels of stress and the impact of the unit-level environment on stress and self-care practices. Incorporating unit-specific interventions to promoting self-care and mindfulness practices is an opportunity to improve nurse stress and promote resilience. Additionally, leadership support is crucial to promoting and maintaining wellness programs.

The importance of self-care at work should be recognized in the workplace by all leadership and considered in budget development. The cost of the 4-week pilot was $10,000, which is a small amount, considering it costs more than $70,000 to train a new staff nurse.[43,44] Using wellness programs, such as Replenish at Work, that are targeted to meet staff needs and are conducted on the unit promotes increased engagement and attendance. These types of programs also can reduce stress and further prevent nurses from leaving the profession due to burnout. Additionally, promoting healthy behaviors among ICU nurses may further translate into decreased turnover and increased work efficiency, which can lead to improved nursing performance and the delivery of high-quality patient care.

FUTURE PROGRAMS

The current study supports the need for further development of meaningful interventions to promote self-care in the workplace to reduce burnout and promote resilience. Finding ways to integrate self-care and mindfulness into the workplace, even in short segments, warrants further research and exploration in practice. For future research, it would be pertinent to refine the program using an experimental design with a larger sample size to allow for analysis of efficacy in other settings. Using validated tools seen in other research projects, such as the Connor-Davidson Resilience Scale,[45] Perceived Stress Scale,[46] and Maslach Burnout Inventory,[47] would further assess comparability of findings. Extending the length of the pilot to include a follow-up period would enable analysis of the lasting effects of the intervention. Additionally, continuing to offer programs at different times to accommodate staff working all shifts would continue to eliminate the need for staff to attend on a day off. Last, focusing on a train-the-trainer method or identifying wellness champions after the intervention phase could further explore the long-term sustainability on the unit level because this has been proved effective in other settings.[43]

Supporting staff through the promotion of self-care and mindfulness is an opportunity to improve nurse stress and promote resilience. Providing wellness interventions, such as the Replenish at Work program for nurses, has the potential to alleviate the immediate stress generated from patient care and provide a moment of peace. The current study supports the need for further development of meaningful interventions to promote self-care in the workplace to reduce burnout and promote resilience.

Within the same organization, work environments can vary. Therefore, future research focusing on organizational efforts should utilize these differences and strive to improve outcomes at the local level in addition to addressing organizational needs. Additionally, more research should focus on the organization's roles in reducing stress by focusing on the improvements of processes and procedures.

SUMMARY

The program outcomes support the feasibility of a brief mindfulness intervention on improving stress levels and promoting resiliency among CTICU staff. A larger sample and more thorough research methodology are needed to further demonstrate applicability. Key takeaways are the reinforcement of the benefit of leadership support in identifying unit needs and promoting self-care. Gathering staff input on barriers to self-care and unit-specific needs should be considered when designing wellness programs. Identifying ambassadors to champion and encourage self-care practices will sustain culture change. Further studies are needed to address organizational improvements of work conditions in combination with individual wellness programs to combat burnout and promote healthy work environments.

ACKNOWLEDGMENTS

The author would like to acknowledge Francine LoRusso, MHA, RN, CCRN, CENP, Vice President of Nursing for the cost center of the HVC and transplantation services at Yale New Haven Hospital, for her financial support in funding this program. Also, the co-facilitator of the Replenish at Work program, Pamela Mulligan BSN, RN, NBC-HWC, RYT 500.

DISCLOSURE

The author has nothing to disclose.

REFERENCES

1. Moss M, Good VS, Gozal D, et al. A critical care societies collaborative statement: burnout syndrome in critical care health-care professionals. a call for action. Am J Respir Crit Care Med 2016;194(1):106–13.
2. Poncet MC, Toullic P, Papazian L, et al. Burnout syndrome in critical care nursing staff. Am J Respir Crit Care Med 2007;175(7):698–704.
3. Rushton CH, Batcheller J, Schroeder K, et al. Burnout and resilience among nurses practicing in high-intensity settings. Am J Crit Care 2015;24(5):412–20.
4. Mealer M, Jones J, Moss M. A qualitative study of resilience and posttraumatic stress disorder in United States ICU nurses. Intensive Care Med 2012;38(9): 1445–51.
5. Maslach C, Leiter MP. Understanding the burnout experience: recent research and its implications for psychiatry. World Psychiatry 2016;15(2):103–11.
6. West CP, Dyrbye LN, Erwin PJ, et al. Interventions to prevent and reduce physician burnout: a systematic review and meta-analysis. Lancet 2016;388(10057): 2272–81.
7. Leiter MP, Maslach C. Nurse turnover: the mediating role of burnout. J Nurs Manag 2009;17(3):331–9.
8. Shanafelt TD, Balch CM, Bechamps G, et al. Burnout and medical errors among American Surgeons. Ann Surg 2010;251(6):995–1000.
9. American Association of Critical-Care Nurses. AACN standards for establishing and sustaining healthy work environments: a journey to excellence. Aliso Viejo (CA): American Association of Critical-Care Nurses; 2005.
10. American Association of Critical-Care Nurses. AACN standards for establishing and sustaining healthy work environments: a journey to excellence. 2nd edition. Aliso Viejo (CA): American Association of Critical-Care Nurses; 2016.

11. Ulrich B, Barden C, Cassidy L, et al. Critical care nurse work environments 2018: findings and implications. Crit Care Nurse 2019;39(2):67–84.
12. Chesak SS, Cutshall SM, Bowe CL, et al. Stress management interventions for nurses: critical literature review. J Holist Nurs 2019;37(3):288–95.
13. Dossey BM, Keegan L. Holistic nursing: a handbook for practice. Burlington (VT): Jones & Bartlett Publishers; 2012.
14. American Nurses Association and American Holistic Nurses Association. Holistic nursing: scope and standards of practice. 3rd edition. Silver Spring (MD): American Nurses Association and American Holistic Nurses Association; 2019.
15. Watson J. Nursing: the philosophy and science of caring. Boulder (CO): University Press of Colorado; 2008.
16. Siebert DC, Siebert CF. Help seeking among helping professionals: a role identity perspective. Am J Orthopsychiatry 2007;77(1):49–55.
17. Thacker K, Stavarski D, Brancato, et al. An investigation into the health-promoting lifestyle practices of RNs. Am J Nurs 2016;16:24–30.
18. McElligott D, Capitulo KL, Morris DL, et al. The effect of a holistic program on health-promoting behaviors in hospital registered nurses. J Holist Nurs 2010; 28(3):175–83.
19. McElligott D. Tag! we're it: holistic nurses as champions for health promotion and self-care. Beginnings 2013;33:10–3.
20. Gillespie BM, Chaboyer W, Wallis M. Development of a theoretically derived model of resilience through concept analysis. Contemp Nurse 2007;25(1–2): 124–35.
21. Medland J, Howard-Ruben J, Whitaker E. Fostering psychosocial wellness in oncology nurses: addressing burnout and social support in the workplace. Oncol Nurs Forum 2004;31(1):47–54.
22. Waite PJ, Richardson GE. Determining the efficacy of resiliency training in the work site. J Allied Health 2004;33:178–83.
23. Montanari KM, Bowe CL, Chesak SS, et al. Mindfulness: assessing the feasibility of a pilot intervention to reduce stress and burnout. J Holist Nurs 2018;37(2): 175–88.
24. Kabat-Zinn J. Wherever you go, there you are. London: Piatkus; 2004.
25. Epstein R. Mindful practice in action, II: Cultivating habits of mind. Fam Syst Health 2003;21:11–7.
26. Lamothe M, Rondeau É, Malboeuf-Hurtubise C, et al. Outcomes of MBSR or MBSR-based interventions in health care providers: a systematic review with a focus on empathy and emotional competencies. Complement Ther Med 2016; 24:19–28.
27. Yang S, Meredith P, Khan A. Is mindfulness associated with stress and burnout among mental health professionals in Singapore? Psychol Health Med 2016; 22(6):673–9.
28. Steinberg BA, Klatt M, Duchemin AM. Feasibility of a mindfulness-based intervention for surgical intensive care unit personnel. Am J Crit Care 2016; 26(1):10–8.
29. Gauthier T, Meyer RM, Grefe D, et al. An on-the-job mindfulness-based intervention for pediatric ICU nurses: a pilot. J Pediatr Nurs 2015;30(2):402–9.
30. Press Ganey. Burnout and resilience: a framework for data analysis and a positive path forward. South Bend (IN): Press Ganey Associates, Inc.; 2018.
31. Sinsky C, Colligan L, Li L, et al. Allocation of physician time in ambulatory practice: a time and motion study in 4 specialties. Ann Intern Med 2016;165(11):753.

32. Linzer M, Poplau S, Grossman E, et al. A cluster randomized trial of interventions to improve work conditions and clinical burnout in primary care: results from the Healthy Workplace (HWP) study. J Gen Intern Med 2015;30:1105.
33. American Nurses Association. Optimal nurse staffing to improve quality of care and patient outcomes: executive summary. 2015. Available at: https://www.nursingworld.org/practice-policy/nurse-staffing/. Accessed September 5, 2019.
34. Kelly L, Todd M. Compassion fatigue and the healthy work environment. AACN. Adv Crit Care 2017;28(4):351–8.
35. Bohman B, Dyrbye L, Sinsky C, et al. 2017. Physician well-being: the Reciprocity of practice efficiency, culture of wellness, and personal resilience. New England journal of medicine Catalyst. 2019. Available at: https://catalyst.nejm.org/physician-well-being-efficiency-wellness-resilience/. Accessed September 5, 2019.
36. Shanafelt TD, Noseworthy JH. Executive leadership and physician well-being. Mayo Clin Proc 2017;92(1):129–46.
37. Yu M, Lee H. Impact of resilience and job involvement on turnover intention of new graduate nurses using structural equation modeling. Jpn J Nurs Sci 2018; 15(4):351–62.
38. Caruso EM, Cisar N, Pipe T. Creating a healing environment. Nurs Adm Q 2008; 32(2):126–32.
39. Sitzman K, Watson J. Caring science, mindful practice: implementing watsons human caring theory. New York: Springer Publishing Company, LLC; 2018.
40. Neff KD, Germer CK. A pilot study and randomized controlled trial of the mindful self-compassion program. J Clin Psychol 2012;69(1):28–44.
41. Siegel DJ. Pocket guide to interpersonal neurobiology an integrative handbook of the mind. New York: W.W. Norton & Company; 2012.
42. Vanhove AJ, Herian MN, Perez ALU, et al. Can resilience be developed at work? A meta-analytic review of resilience-building programme effectiveness. J Occup Organ Psychol 2015;89(2):278–307.
43. Benefits. ANA. Available at: https://nam03.safelinks.protection.outlook.com/?url=https%3A%2F%2Fwww.nursingworld.org%2Forganizationalprograms%2Fmagnet%2Fwhy-become-magnet%2Fbenefits%2F&data=02%7C01%7Cj.surendrakumar%40elsevier.com%7C423c9d5d8a6647c5835e08d812dc4eae%7C9274ee3f94254109a27f9fb15c10675d%7C0%7C0%7C637280085366231955&sdata=2CcezarstaGMSHmkBc9cHNlrslu2EDuA7uNvgrqWDgw%3D&reserved=0. Accessed September 5, 2019.
44. Davidson JRT. Connor-Davidson Resilience Scale (CDRISC) Manual. Unpublished. 01-01-2020, accessible at https://nam03.safelinks.protection.outlook.com/?url=http%3A%2F%2Fwww.cdrisc.com%2F&data=02%7C01%7Cj.surendrakumar%40elsevier.com%7C423c9d5d8a6647c5835e08d812dc4eae%7C9274ee3f94254109a27f9fb15c10675d%7C0%7C0%7C637280085366231955&sdata=vhoAhi6vVw1cDej4gvhD42x%2F8SeDCo5FeSyMe5qN8W4%3D&reserved=0.
45. Cohen S, Kamarck T, Mermelstein RA. Global Measure of Perceived Stress. Journal of Health and Social Behavior 1983;24:385–96.
46. Maslach C, Jackson S, Leiter MP. Maslach burnout inventory manual. 3rd edition. Palo Alto (CA): Consulting Psychologist Press; 2017.
47. Lester PB, McBride S, et al. Bringing Science to Bear: An Empirical Assessment of the Comprehensive Soldier Fitness Program. American Psychologist 2011; 66(1):77–81.

Moral Resilience for Critical Care Nurses

Karen Stutzer, PhD, RN[a,b,]*, Anna M. Rodriguez, BSN, RN, PCCN, CCRN[c]

KEYWORDS

- Ethical work environment • Moral distress • Moral resilience • Moral courage
- Nursing ethics • Healthy work environment

KEY POINTS

- By nature, the work critical care nurses do can lead to moral distress.
- There are evidence-based strategies to successfully address the impact of moral distress in critical care nurses.
- Moral resilience shifts the discussion from one of distress to one of personal empowerment in the face of ethical tension.
- The path to moral resilience requires both personal commitment and organizational support.

INTRODUCTION

Nurses are identified as the most trusted profession in Gallup polls for 17 years in a row. The key contributor to the public's trust is the belief that nurses are honest and have high ethical standards.[1] The American Nurses Association (ANA) Code of Ethics delineates the ethical expectations of nurses as upholding the profession and advocating for the health and well-being of individuals, families, groups, communities, and populations.[2] The expectation to members of the profession is that nurses personally meet the high standards of the profession and the expectations of the public. These stressors are a source of extraordinary pressure on the nursing workforce.

Nurses are often exposed to concerns within their professional environments impacting their ability to act in an ethical manner, resulting in moral distress. There is a professional toll that occurs when one's professional integrity is harmed, resulting in a variety of sequelae for the nurse. Among these outcomes are burnout, job dissatisfaction, turnover, and leaving the profession of nursing.[3]

The phenomenon of moral distress is not new, and it is not isolated to the nursing profession. In examining members of the interprofessional team, including a variety

[a] Nursing, The College of Saint Elizabeth, Morristown, NJ, USA; [b] Thomas Edison State University, Trenton, NJ, USA; [c] Endoscopy, University of Utah Health, 50 N Medical Drive, Salt Lake City, 84132, USA
* Corresponding author. 5 Valley View Court, Newton, NJ 07860.
E-mail address: kstrn1@gmail.com
Twitter: @theburnoutbook (A.M.R.)

Crit Care Nurs Clin N Am 32 (2020) 383–393
https://doi.org/10.1016/j.cnc.2020.05.002
0899-5885/20/© 2020 Elsevier Inc. All rights reserved.

of acute care nursing specialties, respiratory therapists, dieticians, social workers, physical therapists, and physicians, moral distress was experienced by all the participants.[4] When clinicians are not able to care for patients according to their professional ethics, moral injury occurs, leading to emotional exhaustion and disengagement.[5] Developing a capacity for moral resilience may be a path to mitigating the effects of morally disturbing experiences.[6]

MORAL DISTRESS

Moral distress first appeared in the literature in 1984 and was defined as "the psychological distress of being in a situation in which one is constrained from acting on what one knows to be right."[7] Naming the phenomenon opened the door to further discussion of the experience, and the development of a body of literature exploring and addressing moral distress grew exponentially (**Table 1**).

Reasons for this growth reflect an increase in patient acuity and complexity of care, and increased moral distress. Since articulating the definition in the 1980s, the term has become more widely used to describe situations that were previously not given voice to or were defined with different terminology. There is significant prevalence and severity of moral distress in nursing practice, with critical care being a high-risk environment.[8] In 1 study, providers in intensive care units (ICUs) had significantly higher average levels of moral distress than non-ICU providers.[4]

Moral distress is described as emerging in the 2 following phases: (1) the "initial distress" in the moment it occurs, and the action or inaction involved; and (2) "reactive distress," also known as "moral residue," that occurs in response of the initial episode of moral distress.[9] It is important to differentiate the definition of moral distress from other occupational phenomena, including burnout, posttraumatic stress, and moral residue, each of which have their own unique definition.

The main distinguishing feature of moral distress is the "perceived violation of one's own professional integrity and obligations and the concurrent feeling of being constrained from taking the ethically appropriate action."[10] It is important to identify that what is perceived to be ethically inappropriate may vary between individuals, and it often is determined by their preconceived ideas, values, and beliefs.

CASE STUDIES TO CLARIFY TERMINOLOGY SURROUNDING MORAL DISTRESS

The following case studies will help to illustrate the various terms surrounding moral distress and the ethical injuries involved. These scenarios are inspired by real-life

Table 1 Moral distress in literature	
Years (5-y Increments)	Moral Distress Mentioned in Published Literature
1987–1992	13
1993–1998	22
1999–2004	46
2005–2010	173
2011–2016	379
2017–2019 (2 y)	321

(Analysis of the Cumulative Index of Nursing and Allied Health Literature (CINAHL) database conducted October 2019.)

events but contain fictional names and patient information to maintain confidentiality. These case studies are not meant to guide practice, but to act as a tool for education.[11]

CASE STUDY 1: MORAL AMBIGUITY—A LACK OF CERTAINTY ABOUT WHETHER SOMETHING IS RIGHT OR WRONG

Susan is caring for a critically ill, intubated female patient who is newly diagnosed with human immunodeficiency virus. The patient's spouse arrives and wants an update on how his wife is doing. Susan is vague with her response because she is unsure how to respond, knowing the patient is unable to speak for herself and that it is unclear if the spouse could be the source of the virus, or at risk for it. Susan reaches out to the attending provider to help her navigate the situation.

CASE STUDY 2: MORAL INJURY—"BEING UNABLE TO PROVIDE HIGH-QUALITY CARE AND HEALING IN THE CONTEXT OF HEALTH CARE"

Mary works the night shift in a surgical ICU and is assigned to patients in the same area as Joan, another nurse with whom she does not get along.[5] The unit is short staffed, and there is not a nursing assistant available for that shift. Mary delays patient turns and activities of daily living on her intubated patient while she searches out a different nurse on the unit to help because she does not want to interact with Joan. Thinking about this situation after her shift, she feels bad because the patient was incontinent and was not cleaned up as quickly as she would have liked. She noticed that the skin was starting to get red and irritated by the end of her shift.

CASE STUDY 3: CRESCENDO EFFECT—AN INCREASE IN MORAL DISTRESS DURING A PATIENT CRISIS WITH AN INCREASE IN MORAL RESIDUE THAT REMAINS BEHIND AFTER THE CRISIS HAS PASSED

Carlos is the nurse caring for a critically ill patient who develops end organ dysfunction after almost a month in the ICU.[10] During his shift, the patient's condition deteriorates, and after the weekend on-call doctor talks to the family, the decision is made to withdraw care. Carlos spends time during his shift to answer the family's questions about the process and what to expect. The family verbally expresses that this would be the patient's wishes and that they are ready to say good-bye once family from out of state arrives the next day.

The attending provider rounds the next day and provides to the family what Carlos perceives as "false hope"; the decision to withdraw care is reversed, and treatment continues. Carlos and the other nurses in the unit watch this patient continue to decline in a fragile state and began talking among themselves, wondering if they can reach out to leadership to encourage an ethics consult without the primary doctor retaliating against them.

CASE STUDY 4: MORAL DISTRESS—WHEN AN INDIVIDUAL CANNOT CARRY OUT WHAT THEY BELIEVE TO BE ETHICALLY APPROPRIATE ACTIONS BECAUSE OF INTERNAL (PERSONAL) OR EXTERNAL (INSTITUTIONAL) CONSTRAINTS

Bob's patient is confused and nonadherent with her continuous positive airway pressure (CPAP) machine and constantly pulls it off.[10] The unit is short staffed, and Bob is unable to keep running into the room to put the mask back on the patient. Bob requests a patient safety attendant who can sit with the patient but is informed by the house supervisor that no one is available. Bob struggles with the decision to restrain the patient or take a risk and give the patient a break from the CPAP. He reaches out to his charge nurse for help.

CASE STUDY 5: MORAL RESIDUE—"LINGERING FEELINGS AFTER A MORALLY PROBLEMATIC SITUATION HAS PASSED"

Sarah responds to a code gray (combative person) in the ICU and helps to physically subdue a combative patient who is trying to self-extubate while another nurse secures the patient in soft wrist restraints and titrates up on the sedation medication.[10] Sarah feels anxious and shaky because this situation reminds her of a former patient who successfully self-extubated and coded shortly after. Situations like this make her hesitant to perform sedation holidays on her patients even though she knows it is best practice.

CONTEMPORARY DEFINITION OF MORAL DISTRESS

As these case studies indicate, there are a variety of phenomena related to but different from moral distress. In response to further understanding moral distress and clarifying the specific phenomenon, a new definition of moral distress is proposed: "one or more negative self-directed emotions or attitudes that arise in response to one's perceived involvement in a situation that one perceives to be morally undesirable."[4] This definition provides a broader understanding of moral distress and captures all the nuanced interrelationships of ethical tension that can lead to its occurrence.

CONTRIBUTING FACTORS

From these case studies, common themes appear when thinking about the factors that contribute to moral distress. These factors can be separated into clinical causes and interdisciplinary and organizational causes (**Table 2**).

MANIFESTATIONS OF MORAL DISTRESS

Individuals who have experienced moral distress can experience self-doubt,[10,13] can experience perceived powerlessness,[10] and even have thoughts of leaving the profession.[14] For nurses, the following emotions were commonly identified: frustration, anger, worn down/disheartened, fatigue, distress, stress, embarrassment, hurt (that they cannot do more for the patient), increased compassion, and feeling dishonest with families and patients.[8] The most common emotions experienced by physicians included frustration/irritation, annoyance, sadness, guilt, and stress.[8] Other health care providers stated they felt frustrated, guilty, embarrassed, disillusioned/discouraged, angry, worthless/devalued, helpless, and sad.[8] These negative emotions shared between health care workers can take a toll, and those with the highest level of moral distress are those who are in direct care roles (compared with indirect care professionals like physicians).[4]

The ability to measure moral distress was explored to determine the impact of moral distress on health care professionals and to determine interventions that can be implemented.[15] In 2001, Corley's Moral Distress Scale was introduced as a 21-item scale designed to measure moral distress in intensive care nurses.[16] In 2010, the Moral Distress Scale-Revised was developed to be applicable to all health care providers and was used in several studies with good reliability and validity.[8] Changes were made again, and in April 2019, the new 27-item scale was renamed the Measure of Moral Distress for Healthcare Professionals.[15] This latest version represents the

Table 2 Causes of moral distress	
Clinical Causes of Moral Distress	**Institutional Causes of Moral Distress**
Continuing life support, aggressive, prolonged, or futile care that the professional believes is unlikely to have a positive outcome[3,4,10]	Poor nurse-physician collaboration, lack of collegial relationships, poor team communication[4,10,12,14]
False hope given to patients and/or families[4,10]	Working with unsafe staffing levels, inadequate staffing[4,10]
Not having enough time available for patients[12]	Compromised care due to pressure to reduce costs[4,10,15]
Watching care suffer due to lack of continuity[4]	Lack of support from peers and managers in dealing with difficult patient care[12]
Fear of litigation from patients or families[10]	Working with incompetent clinicians[4,13]
Performing treatments that cause unnecessary suffering[15]	Poor job satisfaction[12,14]
	Hierarchies within the health care system[10]
	Policies and priorities that conflict with care needs[10]
	Lack of involvement in decision making[12]
	Years of nursing experience and number of years in current position[10]

most currently understood causes of moral distress and will help guide future research on this topic.

OUTCOMES OF MORAL DISTRESS

Every time a health care professional is presented with an ethically challenging dilemma that harms their integrity, moral residue is left behind.[10] Each morally distressing situation adds to the previous level of moral residue and may result in a crescendo effect, as described in case study 3. Although moral residue is universal, the crescendo effect appears to have greater effect on nurses than on physicians.[15] Other outcomes of moral distress vary person to person, but there are commonalities shared between disciplines (**Box 1**). Learning how to manage these ethically challenging situations takes personal and organizational involvement.

MORAL RESILIENCE

The capacity for resilience has been cited as an attribute that can diminish the negative effects of stressors in the workplace.[17] Resilience is described as an innate force that is present to some degree in all people that can enable the person to cope with and grow from stressful or adverse experiences.[18] The critical care environment gives rise to stressful and morally complex situations, and approaches to mitigate the negative impact are needed. The concept of moral resilience is emerging as an approach in navigating the personal impact of stressor arising when one is faced with situations evoking moral distress. At the heart of moral resilience is the ability of the individual to "sustain or restore integrity in response to moral complexity, confusion, distress or setbacks."[19]

Box 1
Outcomes of moral distress

Job dissatisfaction[3,8,13]

Emotion suppression to not appear weak[8]

Decreased quality of care for patients[8]

Hypervigilant, more focused, attentive[8]

Burnout[3,8,13]

Distancing self from work[8]

Psychological distress[8]

Increased venting[8]

Thoughts of quitting[8]

Staff turnover[3,8,13]

Leaving the profession of nursing[3]

ORGANIZATIONAL STRUCTURES

The nurses' work environment influences the ability to practice with moral integrity. Optimal ethical practice is required in order for nurses to provide safe effective care that is focused on the needs of patients and families.[20] Organizations have a duty to ensure there are structures and processes to support ethical practices and to provide for safe spaces for nurses and their interprofessional partners to raise and address ethical concerns.[21,22] Nurses in clinical practice identified a variety of strategies to promote and sustain moral resilience.[23]

The presence of an organizational climate supportive of ethical practice is crucial to practitioners sustaining moral integrity. Practices exemplifying these supportive environments include creating moral space[21] and assuring access to ethics consultation and debriefing,[24–27] rounds and policies to support discussions of complex care issues,[25,28] and ethics educational opportunities.[27,28]

Organizations effectively creating cultures to support ethical practice assured the resources to support such practice are present. The resources have the full endorsement of the organization and include consultation with knowledgeable practitioners, available around the clock, and staff needs to know that these supports are there for their use.[21] The development of effective resources and skilled practitioners takes time and perseverance.[26–28] The value of ensuring that there is support to address ethical concerns is that it provides organizations with opportunities to improve care and processes and provides clinicians with the ability to effectively retain their moral integrity. The American Association of Critical Care Nurses (AACN), the ANA, and the University of Kentucky provide recommendations and frameworks for the creation of environments that support ethical practice (**Table 3**).

NURSING LEADERSHIP

Nursing leaders in organizations are responsible for the care provided by the nursing staff within the organization. Ethical leadership requires the leaders themselves to demonstrate ethics knowledge and to assure that the environment is conducive to ethical practice. Leaders must foster a culture that recognizes and acknowledges the impact of ethics in the provision of high-quality care.[24]

| Table 3 | |
| Resources | |
Resource	Web Link
ACCN Healthy Work Environment Standards	https://www.aacn.org/nursing-excellence/healthy-work-environments?tab=Patient%20Care
ANA Call to Action Report on Moral Resilience	https://www.nursingworld.org/~4907b6/globalassets/docs/ana/ana-call-to-action–exploring-moral-resilience-final.pdf
American Nurses Credentialing Center	https://www.nursingworld.org/organizational-programs/magnet/ https://www.nursingworld.org/organizational-programs/pathway/
University of Kentucky Moral Distress Project	http://moraldistressproject.med.uky.edu/moral-distress-themes

As individuals, it is key that nurse leaders know themselves and the values that they embody. They must be willing to act with moral courage, acting in accordance with one's value system,[29] in order to successfully foster ethical practice. As stewards of the care provided to patients and as advocates for the practice of nursing, nurse leaders must demonstrate the ability to effectively communicate the values inherent in the ANA Code of Ethics in order to ensure an ethical environment for practice.[29] The nursing culture must acknowledge that ethically distressing events occur, and acknowledging that assistance is needed to address and cope with these situations is not a weakness but an ethical obligation to oneself.

Nurse leaders must promote opportunities for staff to develop their ethical skillset through staff education, debriefing, and interprofessional collaboration. Actively seeking Magnet recognition and embedding the AACN Healthy Work Environment standards into the practice environment can promote nurse empowerment. Leaders must create structures to encourage the process of discussing ethical concerns, such as embedding questions about those concerns into daily care rounds.[25] The ANA identifies policies that can support and enhance the individual when ethically challenging situations occur. Policies to standardize communication, clarify the nurse's role in clinical situations, and identify the process for addressing concerns are crucial.[30]

Nurse leaders can advocate for resources to proactively address ethically challenging situations and to support staff experiencing moral distress. The presence of ethics consultation services, palliative care teams, and chaplaincy services is among the resources that provide positive support.[30] Assuring there are adequate opportunities for educational development for individuals and the interprofessional team enables clinicians to address concerns with confidence.[24]

INDIVIDUAL STRATEGIES FOR DEVELOPING AND SUSTAINING MORAL RESILIENCE

Self-care practices are an effective intervention when building moral resilience. Self-care is so important that Pope Francis spoke about it in his speech for the 40th anniversary of the Catholic Association of Healthcare Workers in May 2019. He said, "The care that you give to the sick, so demanding and engaging, requires that you also take care of yourself."[31]

The act of self-care allows health care professionals to deal with common stressors that come from their professional and personal life.[35] Developing personal strategies to transform moral distress to moral resilience allows individuals to use their strengths to address the negative emotions and feelings of powerlessness. There are a variety of personal strategies one can adopt in order to enhance their moral resilience (**Table 4**).

FUTURE CONSIDERATIONS

Focusing on the individual's strengths and abilities to develop a capacity for moral resilience is an emerging approach to alleviating the negative impact of morally

Table 4 Individual strategies to build moral resilience	
Professional code	• Know and live the ANA Code of Ethics[2] • Know your own moral compass and follow it[23]
Develop moral resilience potential[28,35]	• Know personal values • Develop mindfulness practices • Acknowledge and respect personal signs of distress • Be alert to thought processes/patterns • Remember to pause and reflect • Listen carefully • Be purposeful in developing ethical mindset
Education	• Learn more about moral distress and ethics through forums, Webinars, workshops, conferences, in-person or online education
Healthy work environments	• Engage in being part of change to enhance the environment[24] • Encourage full participation from all colleagues—be attentive to assure all voices are heard • Partner with leadership in the organization to address ethical concerns • Be persistent • Use resources available from AACN and ANA
Support networks	• Connect with colleagues at work when morally challenging situations arise[23] • Confide in friends and family whose opinions you trust • Seek out mentors to give advice[23] • Enlist the assistance of licensed professionals to help you confidentially navigate morally distressing situations (including Employee Assistance Programs)
Emotional intelligence/ assertiveness	• Practice speaking up and being intentional in your conversation[32] • Use communication tools, such as the Situation, Background, Assessment, Recommendation (SBAR) model when communicating with physicians[33] • Embrace advocacy
Self-compassion	• Develop inward, nonjudgmental understanding of your pain, inadequacies, and failures, recognizing you are human[34]
Stress reduction	• Meditation • Mindfulness • Yoga • Reflective journaling • Massage • Music/art/pet therapies
Physical needs	• Healthy diet • Sleep and rest • Time in nature • Physical activity

distressing situations. Little research has been done to evaluate the impact of enhanced moral resilience and its effect on the outcomes of moral distress.[36] The optimal strategies for organizational leaders and individuals to develop and grow in regard to moral resilience have not been well studied. Developing a body of evidence surrounding the developing and sustaining moral resilience capacity beginning during preprofessional education and continuing throughout one's career is vital for the well-being of clinicians and the patients and families of whom they care.

SUMMARY

The aging society, expansion of technology, and rising acuity in critical care environments will continue to pose challenges to the clinician's moral integrity. Assuring that organizational environments and nursing leaders promote ethical practice is crucial to decreasing the presence of moral distress. The Nursing Code of Ethics reminds us that "the nurse owes the same duties to self as others, including the responsibility to promote health and safety, preserve wholeness of character and integrity, maintain competence, and continue personal and professional growth."[2] Advocating for the preservation of moral integrity is an obligation each nurse owes to themselves and to the profession.

DISCLOSURE

The authors have nothing to disclose.

REFERENCES

1. Nurses again outpace other professions for honesty, ethics. 2018. Available at: https://news.gallup.com/poll/245597/nurses-again-outpace-professions-honesty-ethics.aspx. Accessed September 28, 2019.
2. American Nurses Association. Code of ethics with interpretive statements. Silver Spring (MD): Nursebooks.org; 2015.
3. Hiller CA, Hickman RL, Reimer AP, et al. Predictors of moral distress in a US sample of critical care nurses. Am Crit Care Nurse 2018;27(1):59–66.
4. Whitehead P, Herbertson RK, Hamric AB, et al. Moral distress among healthcare professionals: report of an institution-wide survey. J Nurs Scholarsh 2015;47(2): 117–25.
5. Talbot SG, Dean W. Solving the double binds of moral injury. Physician's weekly. 2019. Available at: https://www.statnews.com/2018/07/26/physicians-not-burning-out-they-are-suffering-moral-injury/. Accessed October 22, 2019.
6. Rushton CH. Cultivating moral resilience. Am J Nurs 2017;117(2):S11–5.
7. Jameton A. What moral distress in nursing could suggest about the future of health care. AMA J Ethics 2017;19(6):617–28.
8. Henrich NJ, Dodek PM, Gladstone E, et al. Consequences of moral distress in the intensive care unit: a qualitative study. Am J Crit Care 2017;26(4):e48–57.
9. Epstein EG, Hamric AB. Moral distress, moral residue, and the crescendo effect. J Clin Ethics 2009;20(4):340–52.
10. Lamiani G, Borghi L, Argentero P. When healthcare professionals cannot do the right thing: a systematic review of moral distress and its correlates. J Health Psychol 2017;22(1):51–67.
11. Campbell SM, Ulrich CM, Grady C. A broader understanding of moral distress. Am J Bioeth 2016;16(12):2–9.

12. Budgell B. Guidelines to the writing of case studies. J Can Chiropr Assoc 2008; 52(4):199–204.
13. Epstein EG, Whitehead PB, Prompahakul C, et al. Enhancing understanding of moral distress: the measure of moral distress for health care professionals. AJOB Empir Bioeth 2019;10(2):113–24.
14. Karanikola MNK. Moral distress, autonomy and nurse-physician collaboration among intensive care unit nurses in Italy. J Nurs Manag 2014;22(4):472.
15. Hamric AB, Borchers CT, Epstein EG. Development and testing of an instrument to measure moral distress in healthcare professionals. AJOB Prim Res 2012; 3(2):1–9.
16. Corley MC, Elswick RK, Gorman M, et al. Development and evaluation of a moral distress scale. J Adv Nurs 2001;34(2):250–6.
17. Lachman VD. Moral resilience: managing and preventing moral distress and moral residue. MEDSURG Nursing 2016;25(2):121–4.
18. Grafton E, Gillepsie B, Henderson S. Resilience: the power within. Oncol Nurs Forum 2010;37(6):698–705.
19. Rushton CH. Moral resilience: a capacity for navigating moral distress in critical care. AACN Adv Crit Care 2016;27(1):111–9.
20. Rodney P, Doane GH, Storch J, et al. Toward a safer moral climate. Can Nurse 2006;102(8):24–7.
21. Hamric AB, Wocial LD. Institutional ethics resources: creating moral spaces. Hastings Cent Rep 2016;46(5):S22–7.
22. Rushton CH. Creating a culture of ethical practice in health care delivery systems. Hastings Cent Rep 2016;46(5):S28–32.
23. Stutzer K, Bylone M. Ask the experts: building moral resilience. Crit Care Nurse 2018;38(1):77–9.
24. Storch J, Rodney P, Pauly B, et al. Enhancing ethical climates in nursing work environments. Can Nurse 2009;105(3):20–5.
25. Musto LC, Rodney PA, Vanderheide R. Toward interventions to address moral distress: navigating structure and agency. Nurs Ethics 2015;22(1):91–102.
26. Hamric AB, Epstein EG. A health system-wide moral distress consultation service: development and evaluation. HEC Forum 2017;30:127–43.
27. Grace P, Milliken A. Educating nurses for ethical practice in contemporary health care environments. Hastings Cent Rep 2016;46(5):S13–7.
28. Rushton CH, editor. Moral resilience: transforming moral suffering in healthcare. New York: Oxford University Press; 2018.
29. The practice of ethical leadership. 2017. Available at: https://www.scu.edu/ethics/leadership-ethics-blog/practice-of-ethical-leadership/. Accessed October 19, 2019.
30. Rushton CH, Kurtz MJ. Moral distress and you. Silver Spring (MD): Nursebooks.org; 2015.
31. Hattrup KN. Pope urges health care workers to self-care, avoid burnout. 2019. Available at: https://aleteia.org/2019/05/17/pope-urges-health-care-workers-to-self-care-avoid-burnout/. Accessed October 22, 2019.
32. Epstein EG, Delgado S. Understanding and addressing moral distress. Online J Issues Nurs 2010;15(3). https://doi.org/10.3912/OJIN.Vol15No03Man01.
33. Parker FM, McMillan LR. Less talk; more action: SBAR as an interactive approach for ethical decision- making. Online J Health Ethics 2010;6(2). https://doi.org/10.18785/ojhe.0602.05.

34. Duarte J, Pinto-Gouveia J, Cruz B. Relationships between nurses' empathy, self-compassion and dimensions of professional quality of life: a cross-sectional study. Int J Nurs Stud 2016;60:1–11.
35. Blum CA. Practicing self-care for nurses: a nursing program Initiative. Online J Issues Nurs 2014;19(3):3.
36. Stolt M, Leino-Kilpi H, Ruoken M, et al. Ethics interventions for healthcare professionals and students: a systematic review. Nurs Ethics 2018;25(2):134–52.

Is It Me or You? A Team Approach to Mitigate Burnout in Critical Care

Jin Jun, PhD, RN[a],*, Deena Kelly Costa, PhD, RN[b]

KEYWORDS

- Burnout • Occupational stress • Nurses • Critical care • Storytelling • Teamwork
- Social support

KEY POINTS

- Burnout is a social phenomenon that can be shared among nurses through emotional contagion.
- Current interventions to address burnout focus on individuals and/or organizations.
- These focused interventions fail to address the key aspects of professional identity and human connection that is, fundamental within nursing communities.
- Innovative approaches that incorporate and foster a community of critical care clinicians, such as storytelling, peer-support groups, or expressive writing, could assist in addressing the burnout epidemic in critical care nursing.

INTRODUCTION

Burnout—a result of chronic occupational stress and defined as a combination of emotional exhaustion, depersonalization, and a diminished sense of individual accomplishment[1]—is rapidly becoming a serious issue for health care workers around the world, including nurses.[2] The importance of addressing burnout is more urgent than ever[3]; more than one-half of the 4 million registered nurses[4] in the United States feeling various degrees of chronic job stress and burnout.[5] Critical care nurses may be at especially high risk for burnout and burnout-related conditions.[6] They care for the sickest population in intense environments, managing complex medical care and multiple technologies while providing emotional and social support to their patients and families.[6] The combination of unrelenting stress, heavy workload, demanding physical and emotional environments, and a general feeling of powerlessness can create an imbalance of demand and control, leading to the development of

[a] School of Nursing, The Institute for Healthcare Policy and Innovation, University of Michigan, 400 North Ingalls Street, Ann Arbor, MI 48104, USA; [b] National Clinician Scholars Program, School of Nursing, The Institute for Healthcare Policy and Innovation, University of Michigan, 400 North Ingalls Building, Room 4351 400 NIB, Ann Arbor, MI 48109-5482, USA
* Corresponding author.
E-mail address: jinjun@umich.edu
Twitter: @iamnursejin (J.J.); @DeenaKCosta (D.K.C.)

Crit Care Nurs Clin N Am 32 (2020) 395–406
https://doi.org/10.1016/j.cnc.2020.05.003
0899-5885/20/© 2020 Elsevier Inc. All rights reserved.
ccnursing.theclinics.com

psychological distress.[7] In a study by Mealer and colleagues,[8] 86% of critical care nurses in their sample had symptoms consistent with burnout, 16% with anxiety, and 22% with post-traumatic stress disorder. Thus, burnout is quite prevalent in clinicians, most especially critical care nurses.

BURNOUT IN NURSING

Although critical care nurses are prone to any of the work stress–related conditions identified in **Table 1**, we focus on burnout owing to its prevalence and its potential for substantial consequences on clinicians, patients, organizations and society.

The impact of burnout on individual clinicians and patients is well-characterized. Burnout can have profound negative physical and mental health effects on individuals. For example, burnout has been linked to heart disease, chronic pain, gastrointestinal distress, depression, anxiety, post-traumatic stress disorder, and even death.[9] Even more alarming, a recent study using the National Violent Death Reporting System from the Centers for Disease Control and Prevention suggests that nurses have higher deaths from suicides than the general population.[10]

From the quality and safety of patient care to nurse turnover, organizations are also affected by unaddressed burnout in nurses.[11–14] More specifically, emotional exhaustion—a chronic state of physical and emotional depletion from excessive job stress—has been strongly associated with worsening quality and safety of care. Indeed, greater emotional exhaustion was associated with higher standardized mortality

Table 1	
Definitions of various work-related conditions at work for nurses	
	Definitions
Burnout	Special type of work-related stress—a state of physical or emotional exhaustion that also involves a sense of reduced accomplishment and loss of personal identity.[1]
Moral distress	First discussed by nursing; moral distress arises when one knows the right thing to do, but institutional constraints make it nearly impossible to pursue the right course of action.[70]
Moral injuries	An injury to an individual's moral conscience resulting from an act of perceived moral transgression that produces profound emotional guilt and shame; often present in veterans.[71]
Post-traumatic stress disorder or secondary traumatic stress or vicarious traumatization	Psychiatric disorder caused by exposure to a traumatic event or extreme stressor that is, responded to with fear, helplessness, or horror;" experiencing, witnessing, or confrontation with an event or events that involve actual or threatened death or serious injury, or a threat to the physical integrity of self or others" and involves "intense fear, helplessness, or horror."[6]
Compassion fatigue	Type of secondary traumatic stress that emanates from frontline professionals' "cost of caring" for those who suffer psychological pain.[72] Experiencing compassion fatigue can feel a loss of meaning and hope, in addition to regular burnout symptoms, a person.

ratios,[14] urinary tract infections, and surgical site infections in adult patients.[11] Further-more, nurses experiencing burnout have a decreased level of emotional attachment to their work.[15] In other words, those reporting high burnout have lower job satisfaction and higher intention to leave their organization.[15]

A persistent nursing shortage and increasing health care costs are 2 ways in which society can be impacted by the compounding effects of burnout in nurses. In a study of newly licensed nurses, 17.9% left their jobs within the first year and 60.0% left within 8 years.[16] In the most recent report of critical care nurses, 33% of nurses intended to leave their current position within 12 months.[17] Although the true costs of burnout among nurses is unclear, the related hospital costs (turnover, absenteeism, infections, etc) are estimated to be around $9 billion annually.[18] Thus, determining ways to pre-vent, manage, and address burnout in critical care nurses is of vital importance for nurses, patients, and society (**Fig. 1**).

RISK FACTORS FOR BURNOUT IN NURSES

Although burnout can affect anyone, with or without underlying psychological dis-eases, there are multiple individual and organizational risk factors for nurses. At an

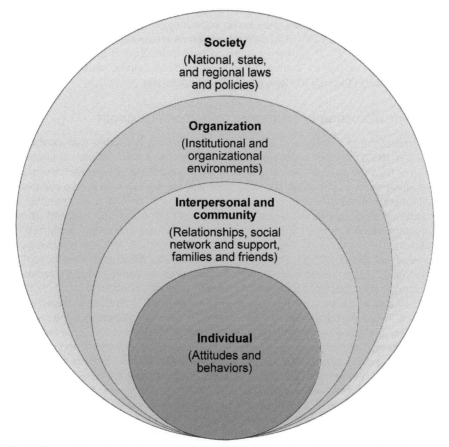

Fig. 1. The social-ecological model. (*Adapted from* Centers for Disease Control and Preven-tion (CDC). The social-ecological model: a framework for prevention. Available at: https://www.cdc.gov/violenceprevention/publichealthissue/social-ecologicalmodel.html.)

individual level, being younger[19] and a woman are known to be associated with increased risk for burnout. In a study by Kelly and colleagues,[20] nurses in the Millennial generation (ages 21–33 years) were more likely to experience higher levels of burnout than their counterparts in the Generation X (ages 34–49 years) or Baby Boomer (ages 50–65 years). Although female nurses reported more burnout than male nurses,[21] how burnout manifests may vary slightly by gender. In a meta-analysis examining gender differences in burnout, women are more emotionally exhausted, whereas men are more depersonalized (or cynical), suggesting that the overall difference of burnout between genders may not be as large as traditionally viewed.[21] Further, organizational risk factors, such as high demands, low job control, heavy workloads, ethical issues, work schedule, and low wages, were associated with risk for burnout.[19,22] Interestingly, key organizational characteristics such as critical care unit type (semiclosed vs open), intensive care unit bed number, long shift lengths, or working on holidays have not been shown to risk factors for burnout in nurses who work in such environments.[23]

Although the individual and organizational risk factors have been well-studied, the role of social and interpersonal relationships at work and its impact on burnout remain underexplored. Positive interpersonal relationships and supportive teams have been reported as a source of great joy in the workplace.[24,25] Thus, social relationships at work, among the nursing team, may be an important yet untapped approach to mitigate burnout, especially in critical care where teams are an essential part of the work environment.[13,14,26,27] To further understand how interpersonal and social relationships could be targeted to address burnout, burnout needs to be understood as a social phenomenon through the lens of emotional contagion.

THEORETIC DISCUSSION OF EMOTIONAL CONTAGION IN BURNOUT

The importance of emotions in organizational behaviors has been well-established since the 1930s.[28] A key aspect of group dynamics and how people communicate and work together is the presence of shared emotions among individuals[29]; the majority of studies only explored emotions at individual levels.[30] Only in recent years have researchers started to examine how emotions transfer among group members,[29] also known as emotional contagion. Emotional contagion has been defined as "the tendency to automatically mimic and synchronize facial expressions, vocalizations, postures, and movements with those of another person and, consequently, to converge emotionally."[31(p5)] The emphasis in this definition is on nonconscious emotional contagion. People "automatically" and unconsciously mimic the facial expressions, voices, postures, and behaviors of others during conversations.[32,33] Contagion may also occur via a conscious cognitive process by "tuning in" to the emotions of others. This is the case when individuals empathize, attempting to imagine how they would feel in the position of another, and, therefore, experience the same feelings.[29]

For nursing, the profession is deeply rooted in human connections and group dynamics. However, despite the long history of exploring and creating connections with patients, nurses' connections with each other at work are often neglected in the research of nurses' well-being. The workplace is where nurses, like most working adults, spend the majority of their time. Today's nurses face ever-increasing demands of work with rapidly changing technologies and more complex care. In addition to the demands, nurses also spend more time working in isolation compared with the previous generation, with electronic documentation and decentralized nursing stations. The unintended consequences of these technologies and rapid changes in care delivery have potentially resulted in increasing isolation among nurses. But the relationships formed at work can be a generative source of enrichment, vitality, and learning that helps individuals, groups, and organizations to grow, thrive, and flourish.[34] Such relationships also can be protective when they develop during stressful situations that are common in critical care settings.[35–37] Thus, group dynamics and shared emotions may play a central role in "spreading" burnout among its members.

Critical care nurses work in close physical proximity to one another. In critical care, there is a significant emphasis on (and need for) effective teamwork and the professional attitude is often characterized by empathic concern.[38,39] These characteristics of critical care nursing are likely to foster a process of tuning in to their nursing colleagues' emotions and emotional state. If more nursing colleagues are burned out, this emotional state may spread among a group of nurses,[40,41] leading to a phenomenon in which burnout is shared across nurses.[18,42,43] Indeed, Bakker and colleagues[18] found that burnout complaints among critical care nurse colleagues were the most important and significant predictor of burnout at the individual and unit levels. Yet, few studies have examined burnout from an emotional contagion lens. As such, few if any interventions focus on shared emotions and its role in preventing burnout. It is plausible that solutions to address burnout in critical could be most effective if they targeted the nursing team, their shared emotions, and social relationships.

CURRENT STATE OF INTERVENTIONS AND POLICIES

As an increasing number of organizations recognize the negative consequences of burnout and its direct and indirect costs, interventions to address burnout have also increased.[39] As shown in **Table 2**, these interventions are often either person directed (individual/groups), organization directed, or a combination of both person and organization directed.[39,44]

Individual-Directed Interventions

Individual-directed intervention programs usually include cognitive-behavioral measures aimed at enhancing job competence and personal resilience and coping skills.[45] Numerous studies examined the effectiveness of individual-based interventions, including mindfulness-based stress reduction, yoga, exercise classes, and/or cognitive-behavioral therapy, art sessions, and wellness activities.[44,46–50] A recent meta-analysis of cognitive-behavioral therapies on burnout demonstrated that these individual-directed coping and stress reduction strategies (eg, cognitive therapies and mindfulness practices) were effective at decreasing emotional exhaustion, but the results were less robust for depersonalization and personal accomplishment.[48,49] Based on the perceived ease of introducing these interventions with promising results, hospitals and other organizations have instituted work-based wellness efforts, such as yoga and exercise programs, and weight loss competitions.[45] However, these programs are often 4 weeks to 6 months in duration, making them a challenge for nurses who are already overextended and hamstrung by scheduling conflicts (eg, night shifts), time spent commuting, administrative burdens, and family commitments.[45,50] Nonetheless, health promotion through workplace physical activity policies, incentives, and supports has the potential to prevent burnout.[51]

Organization-Directed Interventions

Organization-directed interventions are related to changes in work procedures like task restructuring, work evaluation, and supervision aimed at decreasing job demand and increasing job control or the level of participation in decision making.[44] These measures aim to empower individuals and decrease their experience of stressors

Table 2
Types of interventions to address burnout among critical care nurses

	Goals	Interventions (Single or Multimodal)
Individual directed	Practice self-care Practice mindfulness Choose positive	Stress reduction and relaxation training Time management Assertiveness training Work–life balance measures Self-care measures (yoga, exercise) Mindfulness-based cognitive therapy resilience intervention
Organization directed	Reframe nurse burnout as a workplace and patient safety issues Resigning physical and psychological work environments Empower nurses to practice with autonomy (fullest extent of their scope of practice) Engage nurses in designing systems that support their optimal contribution Encouraging managers to support their employees	Promoting healthy work environments Primary nursing model Shared governance Violence prevention intervention Communication training Appropriate staffing Meaningful recognition Schedules
Society directed	Standardize the metrics of measuring burnout and tie improvement to financial incentives Streamline documentations and resources	Policy changes Funding for research

through the creation of optimal and efficient work environments.[44] For critical care nurses, the healthy work environment standards (skilled communication, true collaboration, effective decision making, appropriate staffing, meaningful recognition, and authentic leadership) endorsed by the American Association of Critical Care Nurses[52] are an example of an organization-directed intervention. Since its inception, the evidence of the relationship between the nursing work environment, patient, and nurse outcomes continue to grow.[17] A systematic review of nursing work environment interventions showed that interventions targeting autonomy, workload, clarity, and teamwork made significant improvement in burnout, whereas those targeting communication, management, and leadership did not.[53]

Society-Directed Interventions

Society-directed interventions are ones that focus on improving policy broadly. However, no significant legislative response to clinician burnout exists to date. In response, professional organizations have taken some steps. For example, a call to action was written and published with support from the critical care professional societies, including the American Association of Critical Care Nurses.[54] The National Academy of Medicine launched an Action Collaborative on Clinician Well-Being and Resilience in 2017, a network of more than 60 professional organizations committed to improving workplace culture, supporting clinician resilience, and addressing burnout.[55] The

Action Collaborative aims to raise awareness of burnout while advancing evidence-based, multidisciplinary solutions designed to promote the well-being of clinicians. Professional societies such as the American Association of Critical Care Nurses, the American Thoracic Society, and the Society of Critical Care Medicine have also launched wellness campaigns to decrease burnout and psychological distress in critical care clinicians. Critical care conferences are increasingly adding wellness booths in the exhibit halls, where attendees can receive a massage, pet a therapy dog, or talk with colleagues. Although these are steps in the right direction, additional policy changes at hospitals and even at the state level are needed to address clinician burnout.

Group-Based Interventions Using a Human Connection to Address Burnout

As demonstrated in the review of the current interventions, most are individual and organization directed. Although a combination of individual-directed activities (eg, meditation) and organizational policies changes have been somewhat effective, these steps still do not address the social nature of the problem. More powerful interventions may lie in building relationships among the nursing team owing to the deeply rooted fundamentals of human connection coupled with emotional contagion of burnout. In the following section, we offer several feasible interventions to mitigate burnout in critical care nursing that focus on developing or enhancing human connection among the nursing team.

First, storytelling can be a powerful and therapeutic approach to address burnout.[56] Storytelling is classically defined as the act of an individual recounting an event or a series of events verbally to one or more person(s) with plots, characters, contexts, and perspectives.[57] The procedure of storytelling at work can take multiple forms, but it is with narrative skills and radical listening, storytelling could provide opportunities for meaningful connection with others through personal stories and experiences.[56] Storytelling can also provide a space for nurses to voice their experiences, to be heard, to be recognized, and to be valued, thus improving and humanizing the delivery of health care.[56,57] For example, in a study of storytelling with pediatric oncology nurses,[57] a bimonthly brief informal storytelling session with 2 people, a storyteller and a listener, was implemented. Each person took a turn telling or listening at each session. Although the traditional format of storytelling requires both storyteller(s) and listener(s) to be in the same space as aforementioned study, the use of a digital platform or the process of creating "digital stories" may be more feasible.[58] Although no study of digital storytelling with nurses is published to date, patients who participated in this format of storytelling reported an increased sense of well-being and greater confidence gained through the process of creating their stories of health care.[59] Nonetheless, the format of storytelling is less important than the act of telling and listening to a story. Furthermore, it is important to remember that storytelling is not artificially nurtured through overly contrived and mandatory bonding activities, but rather remains an open and safe space for authentic relationships to develop between colleagues.

Although we acknowledge that storytelling may not be not feasible in certain work settings, peer support groups offer an alternative that have been useful in alleviating work-related stress and burnout.[60] Peer support has been well-established as a beneficial approach for patients undergoing cancer treatment and more recently, for patients after an intensive care unit stay.[61] No 2 peer support groups are the same, but generally they consist of a regular gathering of peers to share their experiences, struggles, and challenges in a safe and close space managed by a group leader to supervise and facilitate the discussion.[60] Although there are some logistical challenges to peer support groups for patients in the intensive care unit,[62] these are unlikely to present themselves for clinicians that work at the same hospital or in the same setting.

Similarly, expressive writing or reflective writing is another potentially effective intervention to extract thoughts and feelings about a traumatic or stressful event.[63,64] For example, the Hunter-Bellevue School of Nursing in New York included a writing curriculum with their nursing students to tell their own stories and to hear their own work and each other's.[65] Critical care journals are also increasingly more open to publishing expressive and reflective writings as evidenced by a powerful essay on burnout by a critical care nurse in the *Annals of the American Thoracic Society* recently.[66] More work is needed to examine, pilot, and research interventions to address burnout by maximizing the strength of the community through cultivating connections and work relationships.

Policy Changes to Address Burnout

As discussed in this article, using a more holistic approach is necessary to address the complex layers of burnout in critical care nurses. A policy or multiple policies on identifying, classifying, and addressing burnout must be included in the overall approach. For example, burnout is now included as an occupational phenomenon in the latest *International Classification of Diseases 11*.[67] Nine European countries (Denmark, Estonia, France, Hungary, Latvia, the Netherlands, Portugal, Slovakia, and Sweden) are even considering burnout as an occupational disease.[68] The Action Framework on the Prevention and Control of Chronic Diseases, deployed by the World Health Organization, typifies this more holistic posture by emphasizing the collection of varied and robust data to identify problematic institutional factors and environmental forces, by directing attention foremost to causes, and by encouraging interventions, implementation, and ongoing evaluation.[69] To be clear, this is not to suggest burnout is itself a "disease"; it is simply to adopt a time-tested and adaptable framework used by experts trained in managing and, ideally, eradicating maladies. Drawing inspiration from the World Health Organization's approach to controlling diseases, while recasting burnout as a preventable rather than simply remediable condition, means proceeding in a more proactive and systematic fashion than we have yet to see in the profession. It requires us to carefully estimate and discern the current need, perhaps through surveys, town-hall meetings, or digital forums, but it also calls for nurses to be central participants—stakeholders—in advocacy campaigns and the crafting of policy, protocols, targets, tactics, and metrics for evaluation.

SUMMARY

Plainly, the status quo for burnout is unsustainable. Risks of burnout are trifold: it affects the individual nurse, and endangers the patients that they take care of, as well as the public that depends on safe and effective care. Addressing burnout requires more than one simple intervention. Fostering human connection to reverse or stop emotional contagion of burnout is what may create the circumstances for nurses to flourish and prevent burnout. To achieve real change, we must reframe the way we view burnout among nurses, as something that may spread among the nursing team and target interventions at the social relationships among the nursing team. Recognizing the contagious etiology of burnout in nurses and the significance of the occupational environment is the first step in addressing this rampant issue among critical care nurses.

FUNDING ACKNOWLEDGMENTS

Funded in part by the National Institute of Nursing Research (P20-NR015331) and the Center for Complexity and Self-management of Chronic Disease (PI: Costa).

DISCLOSURE

The authors have nothing to disclose.

REFERENCES

1. Maslach C, Jackson SE. The measurement of experienced burnout. J Org Behav 1981;2:99–113. https://doi.org/10.1002/job.4030020205.
2. Dyrbye LN, Shanafelt TD, Sinsky CA, et al. Burnout among health care professionals: a call to explore and address this underrecognized threat to safe, high-quality care. NAM Perspectives. Discussion Paper, National Academy of Medicine, Washington, DC. 2017. 10.31478/201707b
3. NEJM Catalyst. Leadership survey: immunization against burnout. 2018. Available at: https://catalyst.nejm.org/survey-immunization-clinician-burnout/. Accessed August 27, 2019.
4. Bureau of Labor Statistics. Registered nurses: occupational outlook handbook. 2019. Available at: https://www.bls.gov/ooh/healthcare/registered-nurses.htm. Accessed August 27, 2019.
5. McHugh MD, Kutney-Lee A, Cimiotti JP, et al. Nurses' widespread job dissatisfaction, burnout, and frustration with health benefits signal problems for patient care. Health Aff (Millwood) 2011;30(2):202–10.
6. Mealer ML, Shelton A, Berg B, et al. Increased prevalence of post-traumatic stress disorder symptoms in critical care nurses. Am J Respir Crit Care Med 2007;175(7):693–7.
7. Karasek R. Job demands, job decision latitude, and mental strain: implications for job redesign. Administrative Science Quarterly 1979;24(2):285–308. doi:10.2307/2392498.
8. Mealer M, Burnham EL, Goode CJ, et al. The prevalence and impact of post traumatic stress disorder and burnout syndrome in nurses. Depress Anxiety 2009; 26(12):1118–26.
9. Khamisa N, Peltzer K, Oldenburg B. Burnout in relation to specific contributing factors and health outcomes among nurses: a systematic review. Int J Environ Res Public Health 2013;10(6):2214–40.
10. Davidson JE, Proudfoot J, Lee K, et al. Nurse suicide in the United States: analysis of the center for disease control 2014 national violent death reporting system dataset. Arch Psychiatr Nurs 2019;33(5):16–21.
11. Cimiotti JP, Aiken LH, Sloane DM, et al. Nurse staffing, burnout, and health care-associated infection. Am J Infect Control 2012;40(6):486–90.
12. Alves DF, Guirardello EB. Safety climate, emotional exhaustion and job satisfaction among Brazilian paediatric professional nurses. Int Nurs Rev 2016;63(3): 328–35.
13. Halbesleben JR, Rathert C, Williams ES. Emotional exhaustion and medication administration work-arounds: the moderating role of nurse satisfaction with medication administration. Health Care Manage Rev 2013;38(2):95–104.
14. Welp A, Meier LL, Manser T. Emotional exhaustion and workload predict clinician-rated and objective patient safety. Front Psychol 2015;5:1573.
15. Chang HY, Friesner D, Chu TL, et al. The impact of burnout on self-efficacy, outcome expectations, career interest and nurse turnover. J Adv Nurs 2018; 74(11):2555–65.
16. Kovner CT, Brewer CS, Fairchild S, et al. Newly licensed RNs' characteristics, work attitudes, and intentions to work. Am J Nurs 2007;107(9):58–70 [quiz: 70–1].

17. Ulrich B, Barden C, Cassidy L, et al. Critical care nurse work environments 2018: findings and implications. Crit Care Nurse 2019;39(2):67–84.
18. National Taskforce for Humanity in Healthcare. Position paper: the business case for humanity in healthcare. 2018. Available at: https://www.vocera.com/national-taskforce-humanity-healthcare. Accessed August 27, 2019.
19. Adriaenssens J, De Gucht V, Maes S. Determinants and prevalence of burnout in emergency nurses: a systematic review of 25 years of research. Int J Nurs Stud 2015;52(2):649–61.
20. Kelly L, Runge J, Spencer C. Predictors of compassion fatigue and compassion satisfaction in acute care nurses. J Nurs Scholarsh 2015;47(6):522–8.
21. Purvanova RK, Muros JP. Gender differences in burnout: a meta-analysis. J Vocat Behav 2010;77(2):168–85.
22. Chuang CH, Tseng PC, Lin CY, et al. Burnout in the intensive care unit professionals: a systematic review. Medicine (Baltimore) 2016;95(50):e5629.
23. Vahedian-Azimi A, Hajiesmaeili M, Kangasniemi M, et al. Effects of stress on critical care nurses: a national cross-sectional study. J Intensive Care Med 2019; 34(4):311–22.
24. Bakker AB, Schaufeli WB, Leiter MP, et al. Work engagement: an emerging concept in occupational health psychology. Work Stress 2008;22(3):187–200.
25. Nurses on Board Coalition. A gold bond to restore joy to nursing: a collaborative exchange of ideas to address burnout. 2017. Available at: https://www.nursesonboardscoalition.org/wp-content/uploads/NursesReport_Burnout_Final.pdf. Accessed August 27, 2019.
26. Halbesleben JR, Wakefield BJ, Wakefield DS, et al. Nurse burnout and patient safety outcomes: nurse safety perception versus reporting behavior. West J Nurs Res 2008;30(5):560–77.
27. Liu X, Zheng J, Liu K, et al. Hospital nursing organizational factors, nursing care left undone, and nurse burnout as predictors of patient safety: a structural equation modeling analysis. Int J Nurs Stud 2018;86:82–9.
28. Brief AP, Weiss H. Organizational behavior: affect in the workplace. Annu Rev Psychol 2002;53(1):279–307.
29. Barsade SG. The ripple effect: emotional contagion and its influence on group behavior. Administrative Science Quarterly 2002;47(4):644–75.
30. Spector PE, Fox S. An emotion-centered model of voluntary work behavior: some parallels between counterproductive work behavior and organizational citizenship behavior. Hum Resource Manag Rev 2002;12(2):269–92.
31. Hatfield E, Cacioppo JT, Rapson RL. Emotional contagion. Current Directions in Psychological Science 1993;2(3):96–100.
32. Bernieri FJ, Reznick JS, Rosenthal R. Synchrony, pseudosynchrony, and dissynchrony: measuring the entrainment process in mother-infant interactions. J Pers Soc Psychol 1988;54(2):243–53.
33. Adelmann PK, Zajonc RB. Facial efference and the experience of emotion. Annu Rev Psychol 1989;40:249–80.
34. Dutton JE, Ragins BR. Moving forward: positive relationships at work as a research frontier. In: Charmine EJ, Härtel CEJ, Ashkanasy NM, et al, editors. Exploring positive relationships at work: building a theoretical and research foundation. Mahwah (NJ): Lawrence Erlbaum Associates Publishers; 2007. p. 387–400.
35. Jenkins R, Elliott P. Stressors, burnout and social support: nurses in acute mental health settings. J Adv Nurs 2004;48(6):622–31.

36. Abu Al, Rub RF. Job stress, job performance, and social support among hospital nurses. J Nurs Scholarsh 2004;36(1):73–8. https://doi.org/10.1111/j.1547-5069.2004.04016.x.
37. Soler-Gonzalez J, San-Martin M, Delgado-Bolton R, et al. Human connections and their roles in the occupational well-being of healthcare professionals: a study on loneliness and empathy. Front Psychol 2017;8:1475.
38. Fairman J, Lynaugh J, Lewensgn SB. Critical care nursing: a history. Philadelphia, PA: University of Pennsylvania Press; 2000.
39. Costa DK, Moss M. The cost of caring: emotion, burnout, and psychological distress in critical care clinicians. Ann Am Thorac Soc 2018;15(7):787–90.
40. Omdahl BL, O'Donnell C. Emotional contagion, empathic concern and communicative responsiveness as variables affecting nurses' stress and occupational commitment. J Adv Nurs 1999;29(6):1351–9.
41. Bakker AB, Le Blanc PM, Schaufeli WB. Burnout contagion among intensive care nurses. J Adv Nurs 2005;51(3):276–87. Neonatal Intensive Care. 2006;19(1):41–6.
42. Nantsupawat A, Nantsupawat R, Kunaviktikul W, et al. Nurse burnout, nurse-reported quality of care, and patient outcomes in Thai Hospitals. J Nurs Scholarsh 2016;48(1):83–90.
43. García-Izquierdo M, Meseguer de Pedro M, Ríos-Risquez MI, et al. Resilience as a moderator of psychological health in situations of chronic stress (burnout) in a sample of hospital nurses. J Nurs Scholarsh 2018;50(2):228–36.
44. Awa WL, Plaumann M, Walter U. Burnout prevention: a review of intervention programs. Patient Educ Couns 2010;78(2):184–90.
45. Jarden RJ, Sandham M, Siegert RJ, et al. Strengthening workplace well-being: perceptions of intensive care nurses. Nurs Crit Care 2019;24(1):15–23.
46. Westermann C, Kozak A, Harling M, et al. Burnout intervention studies for inpatient elderly care nursing staff: systematic literature review. Int J Nurs Stud 2014;51(1):63–71.
47. Kravits K, McAllister-Black R, Grant M, et al. Self-care strategies for nurses: a psycho-educational intervention for stress reduction and the prevention of burnout. Appl Nurs Res 2010;23(3):130–8.
48. Lee H-F, Kuo C-C, Chien T-W, et al. A meta-analysis of the effects of coping strategies on reducing nurse burnout. Appl Nurs Res 2016;31:100–10.
49. Cocchiara RA, Peruzzo M, Mannocci A, et al. The use of yoga to manage stress and burnout in healthcare workers: a systematic review. J Clin Med 2019;8(3).
50. Duhoux A, Menear M, Charron M, et al. Interventions to promote or improve the mental health of primary care nurses: a systematic review. J Nurs Manag 2017; 25(8):597–607.
51. Adlakha D. Burned out: workplace policies and practices can tackle occupational burnout. Workplace Health Saf 2019;67(10):531–2.
52. American Association of Critical Care Nurses. Healthy work environments. 2019. Available at: https://www.aacn.org/nursing-excellence/healthy-work-environments?tab=Patient%20Care. Accessed September 19, 2019.
53. Schalk DM, Bijl ML, Halfens RJ, et al. Interventions aimed at improving the nursing work environment: a systematic review. Implement Sci 2010;5:34.
54. Moss M, Good VS, Gozal D, et al. An official critical care societies collaborative statement: burnout syndrome in critical care health care professionals: a call for action. Am J Crit Care 2016;25(4):368–76.
55. National Academy of Medicine. Network organizations of the action collaborative on clinician well-being and resilience 2017. 2019. Available at: https://

nam.edu/action-collaborative-on-clinician-well-being-and-resilience-network-organizations/. Accessed September 19, 2019.

56. Wimberly E. Story telling and managing trauma: health and spirituality at work. J Health Care Poor Underserved 2011;22(3):48–57.

57. Macpherson CF. Peer-supported storytelling for grieving pediatric oncology nurses. J Pediatr Oncol Nurs 2008;25(3):148–63.

58. Cunsolo Willox A, Harper SL, Edge VL. Storytelling in a digital age: digital story-telling as an emerging narrative method for preserving and promoting indigenous oral wisdom. Qual Res 2012;13(2):127–47.

59. Haigh C, Hardy P. Tell me a story — a conceptual exploration of storytelling in healthcare education. Nurse Educ Today 2011;31(4):408–11.

60. Peterson U, Bergström G, Samuelsson M, et al. Reflecting peer-support groups in the prevention of stress and burnout: randomized controlled trial. J Adv Nurs 2008;63(5):506–16.

61. Haines KJ, Beesley SJ, Hopkins RO, et al. Peer support in critical care: a systematic review. Crit Care Med 2018;46(9):1522–31.

62. Haines KJ, McPeake J, Hibbert E, et al. Enablers and barriers to implementing ICU follow-up clinics and peer support groups following critical illness: the thrive collaboratives. Crit Care Med 2019;47(9):1194–200.

63. Sexton JD, Pennebaker JW, Holzmueller CG, et al. Care for the caregiver: benefits of expressive writing for nurses in the United States. Prog Palliat Care 2009;17(6):307–12.

64. Mealer M, Conrad D, Evans J, et al. Feasibility and acceptability of a resilience training program for intensive care unit nurses. Am J Crit Care 2014;23(6):e97–105.

65. Jacobson J, Jeffries P. Nursing, trauma, and reflective writing. 2018. Available at: https://nam.edu/nursing-trauma-and-reflective-writing/. Accessed October 1, 2019.

66. Leckie JD. I will not Cry. Ann Am Thorac Soc 2018;15(7):785–6.

67. World Health Organization. International classification of diseases 11. 2018. Available at: https://www.who.int/classifications/icd/en/. Accessed October 1, 2019.

68. Lastovkova A, Carder M, Rasmussen HM, et al. Burnout syndrome as an occupational disease in the European Union: an exploratory study. Ind Health 2018;56(2):160–5.

69. World Health Organization. Occupational Health: psychosocial risk factors and hazards. 2006. Available at: https://www.who.int/occupational_health/topics/risks_psychosocial/en/. Accessed October 1, 2019.

70. Jameton A. Nursing practice: the ethical issues. Englewood Cliffs (NJ): Prentice-Hall; 1984.

71. Shay J. Moral injury. Psychoanal Psychol 2014;31(2):182.

72. Yoder EA. Compassion fatigue in nurses. Appl Nurs Res 2010;23(4):191–7.

Igniting Change

Supporting the Well-Being of Academicians Who Practice and Teach Critical Care

Linda Nancy Roney, EdD, RN-BC, CPEN, CNE*,
Audrey M. Beauvais, DNP, MSN, MBA, RN, Susan Bartos, PhD, RN, CCRN

KEYWORDS

- Wellness • Well-being • Critical care • Critical care nursing • Nursing faculty
- Clinical practice • Nursing education

KEY POINTS

- Working as a nursing faculty member and maintaining a clinical practice as a critical care nurse leads to unique challenges and stressors that can threaten well-being.
- Ensuring the environment of those teaching, learning, and practicing within the critical care environment is imperative to the individual's overall holistic well-being.
- Critical care nurses working in the academic environment can implement several strategies to promote well-being.

INTRODUCTION

Nurses are the leaders of patient care, advocacy, education, and advancing the science of caring. Environmental factors such as psychosocial characteristics and interpersonal relationships influence nurses' well-being.[1] The environment also contributes to levels of nursing burnout and job satisfaction.[2] Nurses teaching in baccalaureate programs with critical care faculty or classes in academic institutions may reap the benefits of holistic education and wellness programs and transmit these benefits to emerging practitioners. Optimal outcomes are achieved in the critical care environment when the patient characteristics and nurse competencies are in synergy.[3] The synergy model (**Fig. 1**) is the conceptual framework that drives critical care nursing practice. Spanning the continuum of health, 8 patient characteristics and 8 dimensions of nursing comprise the model (**Table 1**) and can be applied to nursing education. Matching the nurses' competencies with overall patient needs promotes

EGAN School of Nursing and Health Studies, Fairfield University, 1073 North Benson Road, Fairfield, CT 06824-5195, USA
* Corresponding author.
E-mail address: lroney@fairfield.edu
Twitter: @LindaRoneyRN (L.N.R.)

Crit Care Nurs Clin N Am 32 (2020) 407–419
https://doi.org/10.1016/j.cnc.2020.05.008
0899-5885/20/© 2020 Elsevier Inc. All rights reserved.

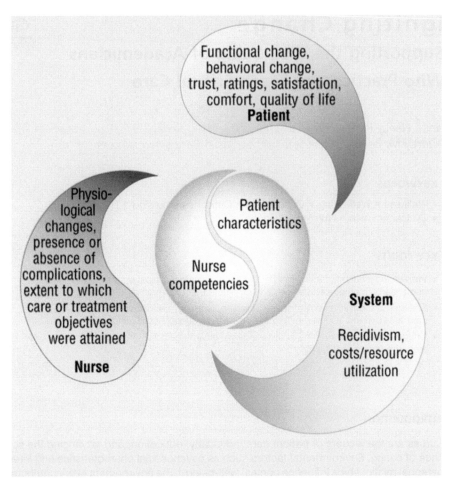

Fig. 1. The synergy model. (*From*: Curley MAQ. Patient-nurse synergy: optimizing patients' outcomes. Figure 2. Am J Crit Care. 1998;7:64-72. ©1998 by the American Association of Critical-Care Nurses. All rights reserved. Used with permission.)

favorable outcomes and supports nurse well-being.[4] This article proposes the application of the synergy model to improve the well-being of academicians who practice and teach critical care. When the student, the faculty, and the academic system are in synergy, learning outcomes improve for both graduate and undergraduate students.[3]

During the outbreak of COVID-19, academic faculty assumed multiple roles as clinicians, academicians, student advisors, researchers, and stewards to the profession of nursing. Because of the diverse clinical roles and responsibilities of academic faculty, varying levels of moral distress were observed. Some faculty were practicing on the front line of the critical care unit and providing direct patient care, whereas other faculty were providing mental health or women's health services. All faculty continued to teach in alternative and adaptive formats and act as a positive representation of nursing to students who will be the post-COVID generation of health care providers.

Application of the synergy model helped to identify areas of impending and active moral distress in practicing critical care academicians. Subsequently, students in both the graduate and undergraduate curriculums faced similar situations. The

Table 1	
Synergy model components	
Patient Characteristics	**Nursing Dimensions**
Stability	Clinical judgment
Vulnerability	Clinical inquiry
Predictability	Caring practices
Resiliency	Response to diversity
Participation in decision making	Advocacy/moral agency
Participation in care	Facilitation of learning
Resource availability	Collaboration
Predictability	Systems thinking

Data from Curley M. Patient-nurse synergy: optimizing patients' outcomes. Am J Crit Care. 1998;7(1):64-72.

importance of a structured wellness initiative emerged to provide support for frontline practitioners in an academic environment. Therefore, this article highlights the use of a structured wellness program designed for those teaching, practicing, and advising colleagues or students in the critical care environment. Strategies for implementing an initiative to benefit academic faculty are shared.

Case Study: Part 1

Robin is a medical intensive care unit (ICU) nurse and an adjunct professor in a school of nursing. She maintains professional certifications and is active in nursing, interprofessional, and educational organizations. Her clinical practice enhances the academic classroom by keeping her material timely, relevant, and evidence based.

During the COVID-19 pandemic, Robin's practice unit quickly transitioned to a designated COVID unit. She found herself putting in extra hours in the ICU while maintaining her academic position and obligations. After a long, 12-hour shift, Robin returns to her home and attends to student emails, lesson planning, and grading. That night, she tosses and turns as the sounds of ventilators reverberate in her ears. She awakes the next morning, returning to her university email before donning her scrubs for another shift in the ICU.

ESTABLISHING THE FOCUS ON THE WELL-BEING OF CRITICAL CARE NURSES
Setting the Standards for Critical Care Nurses

For more than 20 years, the American Association of Critical Care Nurses (AACN) has been committed to creating healthy work environments that support excellence in nursing practice.[5] The "AACN Standards for Establishing and Sustaining Healthy Work Environments: A Journey to Excellence"[5,6] were created in response to a large body of evidence that associated unhealthy work environments with medical errors, ineffective delivery of care, and conflict and stress among health care professionals.[5] These standards include skilled communication, true collaboration, effective decision making, appropriate staffing, meaningful recognition, and authentic leadership.[5,6] Now, more than ever, with the COVID-19 pandemic, these standards are central to the well-being of critical care nurses and those nurses without critical care nursing backgrounds who are charged with caring for patients.

Staffing is a complex process that matches nurses' competencies with the needs of patients, and there is a significant discrepancy at this time. Nurses from all areas of the hospital, often without a background in critical care, are being asked to join interprofessional teams caring for the sickest of patients with COVID-19 with protocols and patient care guidelines that are changing, sometimes multiple times, during a single shift. The stress that this creates for these nurses, who may not have had the desire to ever work in critical care, is significant and can only be matched by the stress of the experienced critical care nurses. Together, this hybrid team of nurses educate each other, minute by minute, on how to take care of the sickest patients in the hospital. With specialty units such as surgical intensive care units and postanesthesia care units converted into COVID-19 medical intensive care units, in addition to staffing, the 5 other standards for establishing and sustaining healthy work environments serve as pillars of support for the well-being of critical care nurses. Positive experiences with skilled communication, true collaboration, effective decision making, meaningful recognition, and authentic leadership contribute to the support that all nurses feel in these settings and to the excellent nursing care that patients are receiving.

To collect baseline data about critical care work environments after the publication of the standards,[6] Ulrich and colleagues[7] conducted an online survey. By this point, more than 50% of respondents were aware of the AACN standards for a healthy work environment.[6] Of particular note, the data from participants showed alarmingly high rates of verbal abuse, discrimination, sexual harassment, and physical abuse by patients, patient family members, physician colleagues, and other health care personnel, as well as administrators, directed toward the individual critical care nurses. Two years later, in a follow-up report,[8] it was noted that there were some improvements with abuse experiences. Ulrich and colleagues[9] completed another survey with samples that were similar in size and representation to past surveys, and the most significant decrease was for the item "RNs are valued and committed partners in making policy, directing and evaluating clinical care, and leading organizational operations" (p 67). Participants also reported feeling less recognized for the value they brought to their organizations, highlighting the need to create healthy work environments and to support the well-being of critical care nurses. In the most recent survey, Ulrich and colleagues[1] found some improvement from the 2013 report; however, most participants reported problems with appropriate staffing, with 6017 participants reporting an alarming number of 198,340 incidents involving threats to their physical and mental well-being. More than half of the participants reported their intent to leave their current position within the year, making it imperative to address the health of the work environment for critical care nurses.

The follow-up data reported the status of the health of work environments before the COVID-19 pandemic. A significant body of evidence supports the relationship between the health of the work environment and patient outcomes and the need to prioritize the improvement of critical care nurses' work environments.[1] Psychological stress, especially vicarious traumatization to nurses caused by the COVID-19 pandemic, should not be ignored.[10] Evidence continues to emerge as strategies to reduce the mental stress of nurses caring for patients with COVID-19.[11] This topic will continue to be a significant area of need as the pandemic progresses, and as the recovery and aftermath of this unprecedented time in history begins and continues for years to come. Immediately before the pandemic, it was suggested that a new type of ICU leader is needed to improve the professional well-being of critical care nurses by using an interprofessional team and a systematic approach to provide vision and improve intractable problems within the health care system.[12]

Countering Workplace Adversity: Is the Answer Resilience?

Workplace adversity can take many forms and harms nursing.[13] Over time, it has been debated whether critical care nurses must develop resilience to support their well-being. Brennan[14] offers that resilience enables critical care nurses to recover, cope with stress, and deal with significant adversities with the expectation that they will "naturally, physically, and mentally bounce back without deliberation activity or attention to the stressor. Resilience, in this sense, is a 'springing-back' process that is meant to leave strong, happy, fulfilled critical care nurses" (p. 281). Nevertheless, well-being and decreased occupational stress have been positively linked to staff resilience initiatives.[15] Jackson and colleagues[13] explored the grounded theory of managing exposure to better understand nurse burnout and resilience in response to workplace adversity in critical care settings. Burnout and resilience are not separate processes but indicators of nurses responding to workplace adversity on a continuum, trying to manage workplace adversity with varying degrees of success. This continuum includes thriving, resilience, survival, and burnout. According to this theory, managing is affected by external factors outside of the critical care nurses' control, such as organizational policies and political climate at the organization.

Empowerment of Critical Care Nurses

The concept of empowerment has been explored for intrapersonal and interpersonal challenges that critical care nurses face related to confronting challenges and feeling powerless.[16] The benefits of empowerment are extensive and include decreased levels of distress and strain, increased sense of control over situation, development and growth, and increased comfort and inner satisfaction. Fitzpatrick and colleagues[17,18] were charged by the AACN to examine the relationship between AACN specialty certification and feelings of empowerment, and to examine these variables related to the participants' intent to leave their current positions. Those with a specialty AACN certification were less likely than those who did not have a certification to want to leave their current position and were more likely to feel more empowered. Concepts central to empowerment in critical care include a mutually supportive relationship, knowledge, skills, power within oneself, and self-determination.[16] Studies support that critical care nurses who have greater access to empowerment structures perceive their work environment as being healthier, and both empowerment and work environment are strong predictors of job satisfaction.[1]

CARING FOR THOSE WHO NURTURE THE FUTURE OF NURSING: HISTORY OF FACULTY WELL-BEING

Historically, teaching in higher education was thought to be gratifying and relatively stress free.[19] Flexible hours, pursuit of scholarly interests, connection with students, and autonomy inherent in higher education were thought to reduce job stress.[20] Over the past 2 decades, higher education has undergone tremendous change that has influenced the well-being of academicians.[20] Faculty face unique demands that may not be apparent to those working outside the role. Job features that once helped to protect faculty from work-related stress are fading quickly.[20]

Recent Trends in Academia

Several trends in higher education potentially influence the well-being of academicians. The first trend is the reduction in funding and resources.[21] University expenses continue to increase, which results in a decrease in the operating budget and a decrease in available resources for faculty. Faculty are being asked to do more with less. Some faculty lines might not be replaced, which may result in increased teaching workloads, increased number of students to advise, and increased committee work. Within the context of the current pandemic, faculty were tasked to immediately transition all of their content to online platforms when universities across the country were abruptly closed because of social distancing recommendations.[22] At the time that this article is being written, there is significant uncertainty about how the fall 2020 semester will proceed on campuses across the country. Colleges across the United States have already suffered significant financial losses from the first 2 months of the COVID-19 pandemic. Future concerns, even if campuses are able to reopen in the fall, include decreased enrollment of new students, including international students, as well as fears that current students may not be able to return because of the economic downturn.[23] Some universities have already furloughed employees,[24] and others are already facing grave concerns of permanent closure.[25]

The second trend involves the changing nature of academic appointments. New faculty often do not have training or preparation in the educator role.[26] New nursing faculty possess the needed clinical expertise but often feel unprepared for the responsibilities of teaching, advising, research, and service. Tenure-track faculty have the added stressful task of navigating the process of tenure and promotion. Tenure-track faculty often cite that they receive little support for creating research agendas and educational skills, an absence of collaboration, and insecurities regarding tenure.[27] If tenure is not granted, typically the faculty member has 1 remaining year in the institution and then must find employment elsewhere. If tenure is achieved, the faculty is expected to continue their growth by showing a record of sustained teaching effectiveness; a record of sustained scholarly accomplishments that have been subjected to peer review; and evidence of leadership in service to the academic community, a learned society, or professional service to other organizations. As a result, many faculty impose excessively high self-expectations that can influence faculty well-being and work-life balance. Over the years, there has been an increase in part-time and non–tenure-track appointments.[21] Faculty in these appointments often have a higher teaching course load, decreased autonomy, decreased job security, and fewer opportunities for advancement.[28]

A third trend potentially influencing the well-being of academicians involves changes in undergraduate education. Institutions are developing programs such as service learning and living-learning communities to assist the growth and development of students. These programs require faculty to teach beyond their fields of expertise and assist students to develop their civic responsibility and develop personal as well as interpersonal skills.[21] Such initiatives require that faculty take on additional responsibilities, collaborate more, and engage in additional activities that may not be rewarded. Another change in education is the increase in technology in the classroom and growth in distance education.[29] This change necessitates that faculty learn new pedagogies, teaching strategies, and learning platforms. Faculty report feeling online teaching is more labor intensive for course development and for instruction time.[30–32] Faculty also report that they have obtained insufficient training and technological support.[33]

Another trend in higher education that influences faculty well-being is the changing student population. Overall, general university enrollments are decreasing, which has led universities to commit to student diversity and inclusion of first-generation, low-income, nontraditional, and minority students.[34,35] The changing student body places additional demands and pressures on faculty as they figure out how to address student needs. Despite general university enrollments being down, enrollment in traditional nursing programs tend to be increasing. Not only have the numbers of students changed but also the mental health of students has changed over the years. Many students experience mental health issues such as depression, anxiety, and substance abuse.[36] Nursing students are not immune to this trend. Nursing students have a tendency to be more anxious and depressed than the general college population as they adjust to their chosen profession and the rigor of their studies.[37] These mental health issues can significantly affect students' academic performance. To address this concern, faculty are expected to identify students at risk and refer students who may be in distress. These personal interactions with students can be emotionally draining for faculty who often feel unprepared to deal with mental health issues.

These trends show that higher education no longer offers the stress-free environment it once did. These trends can lead to faculty experiencing decrease in quality of life, feeling overloaded and emotional exhaustion, which can ultimately influence the well-being of academicians.

ACADEMICIANS WHO WORK IN THE CRITICAL CARE SETTING

Working as a nursing faculty member and maintaining a clinical practice leads to unique challenges and stressors that can threaten well-being. Nurses with dual roles face the challenges noted earlier and more. Working in 2 different roles places extra demands on the nurses' time, making it difficult to maintain a work-life balance. Nursing faculty maintaining a clinical practice have to cope with 2 different job expectations, multiple competency expectations, and heavy workloads. Hence, nursing faculty working in critical care need to be mindful of how to implement and practice wellness strategies. In addition, they have an obligation to teach the next generation of nurses how to properly care for themselves and their patients holistically.

ACADEMICIANS WHO PRACTICE AND TEACH CRITICAL CARE

Ideally, health care agencies and higher education organizations should take a systems approach to professional well-being.[38] The National Academy has recommended 6 strategies to promote well-being: create positive work environments, create positive learning environments, reduce administrative burden, enable technology solutions, provide support to clinicians and learners, and invest in research. Although nursing faculty who maintain clinical practices may have some influence on these system-wide approaches in their organizations, the focus here is on strategies potentially within each individual's control (**Fig. 2**).

Creating the Environment

Critical care nurses working in the academic environment can implement several strategies to promote well-being. For example, they can develop a wellness committee in their departments or schools within the university. At our university's school of nursing and health studies programs, we formed a wellness committee called the Holistic Health Initiative (HHI) with the purpose to provide wellness services to faculty, staff, and students. This initiative assists in threading holistic healing throughout nursing curriculum, including courses with advanced and complex concepts, such as critical care. For example, concepts such as mindfulness, resilience, and reflection are integrated into most of the courses in the nursing major, which helps to ensure that our students are practicing wellness skills so they can competently use them when they join the nursing profession. Another added benefit to integrating holistic healing concepts in the nursing curriculum is that nursing faculty have to be well versed in the concepts in order to teach them to their students.

The HHI has not only revised the curriculum but the committee has organized extracurricular events to promote wellness in faculty, staff, and students. For example, one of our nursing students was trained as a laughter yoga instructor and led a session for students and faculty that was very successful at reducing our stress. The HHI was

PROMOTING WELLNESS IN THOSE WHO PRACTICE AND TEACH CRITICAL CARE

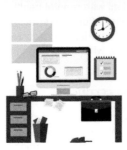

PLAN FOR PROFESSIONAL WELLNESS

- Develop wellness committee
- Curriculum development
- Events for faculty, staff and students
- Seek trust worthy support
- Professional development
- Retreats
- Seek feedback on performance

PLAN FOR PERSONAL WELLNESS

- Journaling
- Maintain physical health
- Sleep
- Exercise
- Nutrition
- Time alone vs time with others
- Self-monitor for signs of stress or depression
- Hobbies

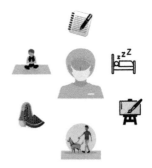

Fig. 2. Promoting wellness in those who practice and teach critical care.

important to establish at an institution with critical care courses and faculty with critical care backgrounds because nurses practicing in the intensive care unit environment tend to have higher levels of moral distress.[39] The HHI convened and served as a resource for faculty throughout the course of the COVID-19 pandemic. Graduates, current students, and critical care faculty within the school of nursing openly shared anecdotal frontline stories pulling the pandemic closer to the individual level.

In addition to establishing a wellness committee, there are other ways to promote well-being in the academic environment. For example, nursing faculty should be encouraged to take advantage of professional development opportunities. In order for faculty and clinicians to flourish, they need to become experts at what they do most frequently.[21] Another wellness recommendation is to seek out trustworthy sources of support. Find mentors who can support you through challenges and opportunities.[21] Developing a personalized wellness plan with a mentor that includes daily meditation and journaling can help decrease stress and burnout.[40] Gratitude journals have the potential to regulate emotion, promote empathy, and provide social reward.[26]

See whether your department can hold retreats. Retreats need not be expensive endeavors and can focus on wellness. For example, at our school, during the COVID-19 pandemic, when critical care nursing faculty were required to convert their face-to-face classes to online formats and stresses were increased, our school planned a much-needed virtual wellness retreat at the end of the semester that include developing self-care intentions, Zumba, charades, and guided imagery. Nurses should seek feedback on their work performance. Many nursing faculty are driven by their desire to excel at their jobs. Thoughtful critique can help inspire nursing faculty and promote their commitment to their role.[21] Nurses should find a trustworthy and reliable colleague to provide them with a thoughtful critic of their work to help inspire them to do better, support them in the work that they do, and leave them feeling committed to their profession and organization.

Physical health (sleep, exercise, nutrition) is essential to well-being.[26] Healthy sleep habits include keeping a consistent schedule, establishing a relaxing nighttime routine, avoiding drinking caffeine or alcohol before bed, limiting daytime napping, and keeping bedrooms cool.[41] Regular exercise has many health benefits, including enhanced mood and resilience.[42] In addition to establishing a regular exercise routine, consider ways to increase activity, such as taking the stairs instead of the elevator. A well-balanced diet can also contribute to well-being and health.

Special consideration has been given by the National Academy of Medicine for clinician wellness strategies during the COVID-19 pandemic.[43] Respecting differences of others in response to the current outbreak is essential; some people find comfort in speaking with others about their experiences, whereas others prefer time alone. Clinicians should self-monitor their well-being for symptoms of stress or depression and seek professional help with any occurrences of symptoms. It is also important for clinicians to recognize themselves and the work of their colleagues during these unprecedented times.

Connecting socially can promote well-being.[26] This connection can take many different forms. Getting together with friends and coworkers outside of work for meals or team-building activities can help build relationships and increase a sense of teamwork when back at work. Starting a book club or another special-interest group can be a useful outlet. Taking time to develop interests and hobbies outside of teaching and clinical practice is vital. Activities such as speaking with colleagues and having hobbies are associated with critical care staff having less posttraumatic work stress and burnout; venting emotion and consuming alcohol are associated with doubling in risk of reporting burnout.[44]

Restoring synergy for both critical care academic clinicians and emerging practitioners in the collegiate environment was a goal of the HHI. Using evidence-based wellness interventions integrated into the student curriculum, the HHI implemented a variety of wellness resources. Support from the institution, along with dually beneficial programming, added to an application of the synergy model to bring together the systematic environment of the collegiate institution, critical care clinicians, and emerging critical care nurses. To be clear, this is not a modification of the synergy model[3] but an application of this theoretic framework to help those who teach and practice critical care. Smaller changes in the academic setting, including music in the office and aromatherapy from diffusers in common areas, can positively affect the mood at work.

Case Study: Part 2

Robin takes advantage of the university's HHI and shares her experiences with fellow faculty. Participating in activities to restore her mentally, physically, and spiritually and bring wellness into her life aid in supporting her through difficult times but also provide her with the personal tools for all times. Robin reconnects with faculty colleagues on virtual yoga sessions and uses humor to alleviate her stress. Although these programs are offered by her hospital, Robin finds it especially comforting to connect to those who are also guiding the new generation of practitioners, sharing strategies on how to manage workloads. Finding solace in solidarity, restoration in purpose in both nursing and education, and approaching her well-being holistically helps pave the paths Robin has chosen to travel.

SUMMARY

Critical care nursing is subjected to especially high turnover rates, with some figures as high as 35%. Ensuring the environment of those teaching, learning, and practicing within the critical care environment is imperative to individuals' overall holistic well-being. With most time spent in the dually dynamic and complex systems of the intensive care and academic environments, it is recommended to implement initiatives, such as the HHI, to mitigate stress, release tension, and promote individual reflections on purpose.

Developing a wellness program to promote the synergistic effect of a healthy work environment for both critical care academicians and students has numerous implications and benefits, such as longevity in the career path, happiness and joy in the workplace, and a sense of fulfillment. Mitigating symptoms of stress and anxiety starts at the hedonic level through programs such as the HHI. Wellness programs are not designed to eliminate sources of stress and burnout. However, they acknowledge and validate individuals' need to self-explore, thereby allowing critical care academicians and students to embrace a true sense of nursing purpose and deliver optimal patient outcomes.

DISCLOSURE

The authors have nothing to disclose.

REFERENCES

1. Ulrich B, Barden C, Cassidy L, et al. Critical care nurse work environments 2018: findings and implications. Crit Care Nurse 2019;39(2):67–84.
2. Copanitsanou P, Fotos N, Brokalaki H. Effects of work environment on patient and nurse outcomes. Br J Nurs 2017;26(3):172–6.
3. Curley M. Patient-nurse synergy: optimizing patients outcomes. Am J Crit Care 1998;7(1):64–72.
4. American Association of Critical Care Nurses. Standards: AACN synergy model for patient care. AACN.Org. 2020. Available at: https://www.aacn.org/nursing-excellence/aacn-standards/synergy-model. Accessed April 28, 2020.
5. American Association of Critical Care Nurses. A journey to excellence, 2nd edition - AACN. Available at: https://www.aacn.org/WD/HWE/Docs/HWEStandards.pdf. Accessed April 29, 2020.
6. American Association of Critical-Care Nurses. AACN standards for establishing and sustaining healthy work environments: a journey to excellence. Am J Crit Care 2005;14(3):187–97.
7. Ulrich BT, Lavandero R, Hart KA, et al. Critical care nurses' work environments: a baseline status report. Crit Care Nurse 2006;26(5):46–50, 52-55.
8. Ulrich BT, Lavandero R, Hart KA, et al. Critical care nurses' work environments 2008: a follow-up report. Crit Care Nurse 2009;29(2):93–102.

9. Ulrich BT, Lavandero R, Woods D, et al. Critical care nurse work environments 2013: a status report. Crit Care Nurse 2014;34(4):64–79.

10. Li Z, Ge J, Yang M, et al. Vicarious traumatization in the general public, members, and non-members of medical teams aiding in COVID-19 control [published online ahead of print, 2020 Mar 10]. Brain Behav Immun 2020. https://doi.org/10.1016/j.bbi.2020.03.007.

11. Huang L, Lin G, Tang L, et al. Special attention to nurses' protection during the COVID-19 epidemic. Crit Care 2020;24(1):120.

12. Hope AA, Munro CL. Leading systems toward improving professional well-being. Am J Crit Care 2020;29(2):84–6.

13. Jackson J, Vandall-Walker V, Vanderspank-Wright B, et al. Burnout and resilience in critical care nurses: a grounded theory of Managing Exposure. Intensive Crit Care Nurs 2018;48:28–35.

14. Brennan EJ. Towards resilience and wellbeing in nurses. Br J Nurs 2017; 26(1):43–7.

15. Babanataj R, Mazdarani S, Hesamzadeh A, et al. Resilience training: effects on occupational stress and resilience of critical care nurses. Int J Nurs Pract 2019;25(1):e12697.

16. Wåhlin I. Empowerment in critical care - a concept analysis. Scand J Caring Sci 2017;31(1):164–74.

17. Fitzpatrick JJ, Campo TM, Graham G, et al. Certification, empowerment, and Intent to leave current position and the profession among critical care nurses. Am J Crit Care 2010;19(3):218–26.

18. Breau M, Rheaume A. The relationship between empowerment and work environment on job satisfaction, intent to leave, and quality of care among ICU nurses. Dynamics 2014;25(3):16–24.

19. Willie R, Stecklein JE. A three-decade comparison of college faculty characteristics, satisfactions, activities, and attitudes. Res High Educ 1982;16:81–93.

20. Kinman G. Doing more with less? Work and wellbeing in Academics. Somatechnics 2014;4(2):219–35.

21. O'Meara K, Kaufman RR, Kuntz AM. Faculty working in challenging times: trends, consequences & implications. Association of American Colleges & Universities. 2003;89(4). Available at: https://www.aacu.org/publications-research/periodicals/faculty-work-   challenging-times-trends-consequences-implications. Accessed April 29, 2020.

22. Anderson N. College students want answers about fall, but schools may not have them for months. Education. 2020. Available at: https://www.washingtonpost.com/local/education/will-colleges- reopen-in-the-fall-coronavirus-crisis-offers-only-hazy-scenarios/2020/04/22/a124edae-83d3-11ea-ae26-989cfce1c7c7_story.html.   Accessed April 28, 2020.

23. Binkley C, Amy J. Financial hits pile up for colleges during pandemic as some fight to survive. Pittsburgh Post-Gazette. 2020. Available at: https://www.postgazette.com/news/education/2020/04/07/Financial-hits-university-college-lose-money-fight-to-survive-pandemic-COVID-19/stories/202004070070. Accessed April 28, 2020.

24. Kelderman E. Major cost-cutting begins in response to covid-19, with faculty and staff furloughs and pay cuts. The chronicle of higher education 2020. Available at: https://www.chronicle.com/article/major-cost-cutting-begins-in/248558.   Accessed April 30, 2020.

25. Rathke L. Virus and Vermont: colleges board weighs closing 3 campuses. U.S. News & world report. Available at: https://www.usnews.com/news/best-states/

vermont/articles/2020-04-20/virus-and-vermont-college-board-weighs-closing-3-campuses. Accessed April 30, 2020.

26. Owens J, Kottwitz C, Tiedt J, et al. Strategies to attain faculty work-life balance. Available at: https://library.osu.edu/ojs/index.php/BHAC/article/viewFile/6544/5113. Accessed April 30, 2020.

27. Eagan MK, Stolzenber EB, Lorzano J, et al. Undergraduate teaching faculty: the HERI faculty survey. Available at: https://www.heri.ucla.edu/monographs/HERI-FAC2017-monograph.pdf. Accessed April 30, 2020.

28. Ott M, Cisneros J. Understanding the changing faculty workforce in higher education: a comparison of non-tenure track and tenure line experiences. Educ Policy Anal Arch 2015;23(90):90.

29. Allen IE, Seamen J. Grade change: tracking online education in the United States. Available at: https://www.onlinelearningsurvey.com/reports/gradechange.pdf. Published2014. Accessed April 28, 2020.

30. Allen IE, Seamen J. Learning on demand: online education in the United States 2009. Available at: https://files.eric.ed.gov./fulltext/ED529931.pdf. Accessed April 28, 2020.

31. Chiasson K, Terras K, Smart K. Faculty perceptions of moving a face-to-face course to online instruction. Journal of College Teaching & Learning (TLC) 2015;12(4):231–40.

32. Merillat L, Scheibmeir M. Developing a quality improvement process to optimize faculty success. Online Learning 2016;20(3):159–72. Available at: https://doi.org/10.24059/olj.v20i3.977. Accessed April 13, 2020.

33. Seirup HJ, Tirotta R, Blue E. Online education: panacea or plateau. Journal for Leadership and Instruction 2016;15(1):5–8. Available at: https://files.eric.ed.gov/fulltext/EJ1097549.pdf.

34. Bransberger P, Michelau DK. Knocking on the college door: projections of high school graduates. Boulder (CO): Western Interstate Commission for Higher Education; 2016. Available at: https://knocking.wiche.edu/reports/privates.

35. Hainline L, Gaines M, Long Feather C, et al. Changing students, faculty and institutions in the twenty-first century. Peer Rev 2010;12(3):7–15. Available at: https://aacu.org/publications-research/periodicals/changing-students-faculty-and-institutions-twenty-first-century.

36. Roy N. The rise of mental health on college campuses: protecting the emotional health of our nation's college students. Higher Education Today 2018. Available at: https://www.higheredtoday.org/2018/12/17/rise-mental-health-college-campuses-protecting-emotional-health-nations-college-students/. Accessed April 14, 2020.

37. Rathnayake S, Ekanayaka J. Depression, anxiety and stress among undergraduate nursing students in a public university in Sri Lanka. Int J Caring Sci 2016;9(3):1020–32.

38. National Academy of Medicine. Taking action against clinician burnout: a systems approach to professional well-being 2019. Available at: https://www.nap.edu/catalog/25521/taking-action-against-clinician-burnout-a-systems- approach-to-professional.

39. McAndrew NS, Leske J, Schroeter K. Moral distress in critical care nursing: the state of the science. Nurs Ethics 2018;25(5):552–70.

40. Chung AS, Felber R, Han E, et al. A targeted mindfulness curriculum for medical students during their emergency medicine clerkship experience. West J Emerg Med 2018;19(4):762–6.

41. Centers for Disease Control. Are you getting enough sleep? Centers for disease control and prevention. 2020. Available at: https://www.cdc.gov/sleep/features/getting-enough-sleep.html. Accessed April 30, 2020.
42. Cotman CW, Berchtold NC, Christie LA. Exercise builds brain health: key roles of growth factor cascades and inflammation [published correction appears in Trends Neurosci. 2007 Oct;30(10):489]. Trends Neurosci 2007;30(9):464–72.
43. National Academy of Medicine. The National Academies are responding to the COVID-19 pandemic. 2020. Available at: https://nam.edu/initiatives/clinician-resilience-and-well- being/clinician-well-being-strategies-during-covid-19/. Accessed April 30, 2020.
44. Colville GA, Smith JG, Brierley J, et al. Coping with staff burnout and work-related posttraumatic stress in intensive care. Pediatr Crit Care Med 2017;18(7):e267–73.

Self-Care in the Bereavement Process

Jennifer L. McAdam, PhD, RN[a],*, Alyssa Erikson, PhD, RN[b,1]

KEYWORDS

- Bereavement • End-of-life care • Compassion fatigue • Moral distress • Self-care
- Critical care nursing

KEY POINTS

- Critical care nurses experience end-of-life and bereavement care on a recurring basis.
- Providing end-of-life and bereavement care can lead to negative physical and psychological consequences for critical care nurses, such as compassion fatigue and burnout.
- Self-care focusing on the physical, emotional, and spiritual aspects is an essential consideration for promoting the health and well-being of critical care nurses who provide end-of-life and bereavement care.
- Healthy work environments and authentic leaders are integral in promoting self-care in the workplace.

INTRODUCTION

Critical care nurses frequently provide end-of-life and bereavement care. Although this type of care is rewarding, it can also put the nurse at risk for moral distress, compassion fatigue, and burnout. By incorporating self-care into their routine, critical care nurses can minimize this risk and maintain their own health and well-being. But how can critical care nurses readily incorporate self-care techniques into their practice?

The purpose of this literature review is to provide suggestions for promoting physical, emotional, and spiritual self-care for nurses who are caring for dying intensive care unit patients and their families. We use a case scenario to help illustrate the importance of this concept. In addition, we highlight practical examples of self-care and discuss how leadership can best support self-care and maintain a healthy work environment.

[a] Nursing, Samuel Merritt University, Oakland, CA, USA; [b] Nursing, California State University, Monterey Bay, Monterey, CA, USA
[1] Present address: 100 Campus Center Drive, Seaside, CA 93955.
* Corresponding author. 1720 S. Amphlett Blvd, Suite 300, San Mateo, CA 94402.
E-mail address: jmcadam@samuelmerritt.edu

Crit Care Nurs Clin N Am 32 (2020) 421–437
https://doi.org/10.1016/j.cnc.2020.05.005
0899-5885/20/© 2020 Elsevier Inc. All rights reserved.

CASE SCENARIO

Kathy is a 29-year-old critical care nurse who has been working the night shift in an adult medical-surgical unit for the last 5 years. The past 2 months have been particularly stressful because the unit had a higher than average number of patient deaths. Lately, Kathy has felt a lack of energy at work, where she often feels unsupported. "It seems like all I do is take care of dying patients. And then before I have a chance to process anything, I have to move on and care for another patient. I don't think the nurse manager and the physicians are as helpful as they could be. They often give the family false hope and expect us nurses to pick up the pieces." Kathy has discussed with a close friend that she is uncertain she can continue her job. She feels burned out and is even thinking about leaving the profession.

BEREAVEMENT IS AN ISSUE TO THE CRITICAL CARE NURSE'S WELL-BEING

Nurses of adult critical care units experience high mortality rates,[1] and they are the ones who routinely provide most aspects of end-of-life and bereavement care.[2,3] This can encompass assisting with family care conferences and decision-making, to managing symptoms, to performing postmortem care, to following up with families after the death.[4,5] Many of these end-of-life situations are fraught with ethical implications and can lead to physical and psychological repercussions for the nurse.[6,7] In addition, the hectic pace of the intensive care unit environment and workload expectations leave minimal time for the nurse to emotionally process the death of their patients.[8] Their feelings often go unrecognized. In addition, they may have little to no formal training in strategies on how to deal with their feelings and grief.[6] The moral distress around providing end-of-life and bereavement care may be a major reason that nurses consider leaving the profession.[9]

THE EMOTIONAL TOLL OF GRIEF

In recent years, research on providing quality end-of-life and bereavement care to patients and their families has garnered much attention and education.[10–12] But an often neglected area is how the end-of-life experience affects critical care nurses.[3] There are tacit expectations that nurses must suppress their grief, hide their feelings, and go back to work caring for another patient.[6,13] Expressions of grief may be seen as unprofessional, selfish, or even as a sign of weakness.[6,8,14] A comment from Kathy highlights this:

> There's not really anything to help nurses…Last night, I spent all shift with this patient, Georgia. She finally died at 5:00 AM - and it wasn't a good death. She died in pain with her family arguing about the best course of care for her. Then, it was not even 10 minutes after Georgia died that I was told that I was getting an admission from the emergency department. I had no time to process anything. I just had to suck it up. At the end of my shift, I went home and that's it. Just a horrible situation to be in.

Critical care nurses like Kathy routinely deal with death and dying, which results in an emotional toll.[3,15] Increased exposure to sudden patient deaths, prolonged dying patients, and actively grieving families can leave nurses overwhelmed with their own feelings of grief and loss.[6,7] Unresolved multiple episodes of grief can lead to cumulative grief.[16] This type of grief can have negative consequences for the nurse's professional and personal life. Cumulative grief has been associated with an increase in occupational stress, moral distress, anxiety, depression, suicidal thoughts, physical illness, substance abuse, poor self-esteem, and even burnout and compassion fatigue in critical care professionals.[3,5,16–20] These issues are then associated with suboptimal patient care, such as disengagement, increase in medical errors, and absenteeism, and may be the major reason that many leave critical care.[3,19]

INDIVIDUAL NURSE RISK FACTORS, ARE YOU AT RISK?

There are several risk factors that are associated with an increase in moral distress, compassion fatigue, and burnout in critical care nurses. Early recognition allows the nurse to develop appropriate self-care strategies to lessen the burden of these factors. These risk factors include:

- Personality factors (eg, feeling the need to always be perfect, having traits of neuroticism)[21]
- Demographic factors (eg, younger age of the nurse, being single, being childless)[21]
- Work-related factors (eg, dealing with end-of-life and ethical issues, less years of experience as a nurse, working the night shift, heavy workload, unsupportive hospital/unit culture)[21]

For example, in Kathy's case, we can identify several risk factors that put her at an increased risk of moral distress, burnout, and compassion fatigue. These include being younger in age, dealing with end-of-life and ethical issues, not feeling supported at work, and working the night shift.

WHAT IS SELF-CARE AND WHY IS IT IMPORTANT DURING BEREAVEMENT?

Broadly speaking, the definition of self-care consists of the conscious practice of caring for oneself. It is the ability to perform the necessary activities to achieve, maintain, and promote optimal physical and mental health.[22,23] Practicing self-care is an occupational responsibility for nurses dealing with end-of-life and bereavement care. Grief, because of its dynamic, pervasive, and individualized nature,[6] is considered an occupational hazard. It may affect critical care nurses physically, emotionally, and spiritually.[24] Therefore, the nurse needs to be introspective on how they feel about death and dying. They need to understand how these deaths affect their overall well-being and how to best take care of themselves.[5]

Adequate self-care is vital to the nurses' own health as it is to providing compassionate end-of-life care to patients and their families. It is important nurses gain awareness of their needs and develop strategies to improve self-care. Next is a discussion of techniques that critical care nurses, such as Kathy, can use to improve self-care.

SELF-CARE PLAN FOR NURSES

- Develop awareness and use self-care techniques from each of the following domains:
  - Physical
  - Emotional and cognitive
  - Personal and professional relationships
  - Spiritual

DEVELOPING AWARENESS USING A SELF-INVENTORY

The first step in practicing self-care is developing awareness. Awareness is the act of becoming consciously alert to one's physical, cognitive, and emotional reactions to challenging or stressful situations.[25] The best way to develop awareness is to complete a self-inventory. Self-inventory techniques vary widely, so we highlight two practical examples:

1. A challenging situation inventory
2. An as-needed basis inventory

The first type of self-inventory is designed to be completed during a challenging situation, such as providing end-of-life care (**Box 1**).[25] For example, Kathy could have used this inventory when she was caring for Georgia. She could take a moment to answer the questions in the inventory in **Box 1** and assess how she was feeling during her shift. This would allow her to recognize her physical responses (eg, tense shoulders and headache) and emotional responses (eg, stress and anger) to the situation. Kathy can learn to identify her responses and act proactively (eg, practice deep breathing) rather than reactively (eg, anger toward a physician or coworker).[25]

The second type of self-inventory is designed to be completed on an as-needed basis (**Box 2**).[26,27] Using this type of inventory can help a nurse recognize when they may be suffering from burnout or compassion fatigue[18] and are in need of self-care or in need of enhancing their self-care. For example, after a particularly difficult week or month where Kathy experienced many deaths, she could complete this type of inventory to check-in with how she is coping and reflect on her need for additional self-care techniques.[8]

DEVELOPING A SELF-CARE PLAN

Critical care nurses often feel selfish when taking time to care for themselves.[6] Self-care is a delicate balance between providing compassionate care for others and yourself. Routinely practicing self-care can help achieve positive outcomes, such as

---

Box 1
Questions to ask during a self-inventory

Physical
- What are my physical reactions to feeling upset?
- Does my stomach tense or do I feel nauseated?
- Do I feel like hitting someone or something?
- What part of my body gets tense (shoulders, neck, back)?
- Do I have difficulty breathing or difficulty catching my breath?

Cognitive
- What are my thoughts?
- Is there one thought about a person or situation or myself that stands out?
- What is this thought telling me about this person, the situation, or myself?

Emotions
- What is my emotional reaction to the situation?
- How am I feeling about the situation?
- Do I feel a lack of purpose?

Spirit
- What caused me to question or abandon my core values?
- How am I really viewing this person, the situation, and myself?
- What are the ways I can learn from this so my peace and joy are not affected?

From Crane PJ, Ward SF. Self-healing and self-care for nurses. AORN J. 2016;104(5):390; with permission.

Box 2
Routine self-care inventory to check in with your well-being

If any of these pertain to you, it is time to practice self-care:
- Do you feel exhausted or more tired than usual after your shift in the intensive care unit?
- Lately have you had more trouble falling asleep or staying asleep?
- Do you constantly worry or feel anxious when thinking about caring for the patients on your unit?
- Are you suffering from problems, such as anxiety, depression, or irritability?
- Do you find yourself frequently questioning the choices you made during your shift and see how they could have gone differently?
- Are you less sympathetic toward your patients and their families?
- Do family or friends share concerns with you that you take your work home with you?

Data from Caffrey PM. A gentle reminder to make time for yourself. Available at: https://www. calvaryhospital.org/self-care-for-palliative-care-professionals/. Accessed October 7th, 2019; and Dyrbye LN, Johnson PO, Johnson LM, et al. Efficacy of the well-being index to identify distress and well-being in U.S. nurses. Nurs Res. 2018;67(6):447–55.

---

finding joy and comfort and to help build resiliency.[28] When developing a self-care plan, the suggestion is to try to incorporate and practice one activity or technique daily from each domain and then add more as needed. In addition, enlisting the help of a colleague can provide accountability and emotional support.

PHYSICAL BODY SELF-CARE TECHNIQUES

Physical responses to grief commonly include such issues as stomachaches, nausea, headaches, and a general feeling of being unwell.[24,29] In addition, the body typically responds to stressful events by activating the sympathetic nervous system. With this response, blood pressure goes up, heart rate increases, muscle tenses, breathing becomes shallow, and cortisol levels rise.[29] Practicing techniques that initiate the parasympathetic nervous system can mitigate these responses by slowing down the heart rate and lowering the blood pressure. There are many studies that support the effectiveness and benefits of physical techniques in helping reduce the physical effects of grief on the body.[25,30] For example, the next time Kathy is feeling overwhelmed at work, she could try a deep breathing exercise. She first finds somewhere private where she can sit down. She then places one hand over her chest and the other hand over her abdomen. As she breaths in deeply she repeats the phrase, "I am in control." And as she exhales, she repeats, "I am blowing away my stress." This technique has the advantage of being practiced quickly and can bring the body back into balance. **Table 1** provides additional suggestions and descriptions of physical self-care techniques that the critical care nurse can practice to help alleviate grief and stress when providing end-of-life and bereavement care.[8,23,25,31,32]

EMOTIONAL AND COGNITIVE SELF-CARE TECHNIQUES

Emotional responses to grief often include such behaviors as increased irritability; anxiety; numbness; self-doubt; or practicing unhealthy behaviors, such as drinking or overeating.[24,25,33] In addition, emotional responses are typically triggered by our frame of mind.[34] Learning to choose thoughts that support self-care are necessary to the health and well-being of the critical care nurse. Examining how to break patterns of thought can result in a greater emotional balance. When Kathy felt helpless taking care of Georgia, she had these thoughts: *I can't do anything for this patient, no matter*

Table 1
Physical self-care techniques

Type	Benefits	Suggestions and Examples
Deep breathing exercises	Consciously slowing down your breathing helps bring the physical responses back into balance	Place one hand at the top of the chest and one hand over the abdomen Practice breathing so that the hand over the abdomen moves first Exhale for twice as long as it takes to inhale This can be completed seated or laying down
Body awareness	This technique is useful for bringing awareness of sensations before they become tense or painful in the body	This technique requires 30–60 s and can be practiced throughout the day Close eyes and take a few deep breaths Start at the top of the head, become aware of the sensations of the head, neck, and shoulders Continue to assess moving down the body sensing which parts feel tense and which parts feel relaxed Focus on the parts that feel relaxed and imagine that relaxation spreading to all parts of the body
Relaxation exercises and Progressive relaxation exercises	This technique helps enhance the body's relaxation response and teaches the body how to respond to verbal commands	Practice tensing muscle groups and then releasing them to recognize the difference in those sensations
Meditation	Mindfulness technique that lowers blood pressure, improves focus and attention, and decreases depression Many nurses feel they do not have the time for this during their shift; it does not need to be 10–20 min (although that is ideal)	Find a quiet place Consciously relax the body's muscles Focus for 10–20 min (if possible) on a specific word or phrase Assume a passive attitude toward intrusive thoughts
Exercise	Lowers blood pressure and blood sugar levels Improves endorphins and overall physical fitness Help improve cognition and emotions	Take short walks during a break Get an app or device that tracks your steps Practice yoga poses Aim for 150 min of moderate aerobic activity per week along with 2 d of strengthening exercises for the most benefit

Nutrition	Decreases risk of chronic disease and obesity	Eat more nutrient-dense vegetables, whole grains, fruits, low-fat dairy, proteins, and healthy oils
		Limit the amount of sugar, fats, and salt in the diet
		Try to minimize poor eating habits (eg, rushed eating, junk food)
		Advocate for healthier options at the cafeteria
		Try to obtain a refrigerator for the unit to bring in healthier food from home
		Inquire if vending machines can offer healthier food
Sleep	Helps the body and mind rejuvenate and helps maintain good overall health	7 or more hours of sleep in a 24-h period is recommended
	May help enhance productivity, cognitive functioning, and lower risk of chronic diseases (eg, diabetes, heart disease)	

Data from Refs.[8,23,25,31,32]

what I do, she will not survive. Instead Kathy could practice changing her thinking to, *I am doing the best I can and I can help Georgia be comfortable and her family feel supported.* **Box 3** provides further examples of positive self-talk.[25,35]

Providing care to dying patients is emotionally challenging and causes strong reactions. This may bring up significant events involving loss in the nurses' past. The key to emotional self-care is to acknowledge and process these thoughts, reactions, and feelings of grief and then to release them.[28] It is important for nurses to reflect on what will help them deal with emotional issues. For example, Kathy could practice a soothing outlet, such as taking a hot bath after work to "wash away the day." **Table 2** lists several strategies that critical care nurses can practice to enhance their emotional and cognitive self-care during end-of-life and bereavement care.[6,7,14,19,23,25,28,36–46]

PERSONAL AND PROFESSIONAL RELATIONSHIPS SELF-CARE TECHNIQUES

This self-care domain refers to the ability to maintain relationships and interpersonal connections to others, such as family, friends, and colleagues.[23] These are the type of relationships that enhance our lives. The nurse turns to these people for support during difficult times. Because working with dying patients is physically and emotionally demanding, having a strong support system is essential. One study discussed the power of informal debrief groups versus formal debrief groups in helping nurses feel supported.[8] For example, Kathy could invite a coworker out for coffee where they could share their experiences and help each other through challenging times at work. **Table 3** discusses additional techniques and strategies the critical care nurse can incorporate to enhance their personal and professional self-care.[7,8,23,28,36,47]

SPIRITUAL SELF-CARE TECHNIQUES

Enhancing one's spiritual self-care allows the nurse to search for meaning and purpose in their life.[23] However, it is easy to lose the spiritual aspect of self-care especially when providing end-of-life care. This work is burdened with minutia, policies, details, and paperwork. This may limit time for spiritual self-renewal.[3] Developing spiritual self-care techniques allows nurses to create a sense of peace and a sense of purpose and place in the world.[28] Cultivating a spiritual perspective may have the power to restore

---

Box 3
Examples of positive self-talk

- I have the power to change my mind
- It is okay if I am not perfect
- I am capable and strong and I want to improve my physical and mental health for me
- This is a wonderful opportunity for me to learn from my coworkers
- I can handle a situation even if it does not go my way
- I do not need to take this comment or situation personally
- I can choose not to engage in conflict

Data from Crane PJ, Ward SF. Self-healing and self-care for nurses. AORN J. 2016;104(5):386–400; and Scott E. Reduce stress and improve your life with positive self talk. Available at: https://www.verywellmind.com/how-to-use-positive-self-talk-for-stress-relief-3144816. Accessed October 24, 2019.

Table 2
Emotional and cognitive self-care techniques

Type	Benefit	Suggestions and Examples
Mindfulness Techniques may include: Body scanning Meditation Mindfulness yoga Mindfulness-based stress reduction	Ability to maintain awareness moment-by-moment of one's thoughts, feelings, and body sensations Associated with fewer physical and psychological symptoms, lower stress, reduced exhaustion, and improved self-compassion	Recommendation is to practice some type of mindfulness strategy 10–30 min daily One suggestion is to integrate a 5-min mindfulness session before shift change Another suggestion is to hold 1-h weekly group mindfulness sessions on the unit at a convenient time for most staff
CBT and resiliency training	A useful tool for critical care nurses because they work in a setting with exposure to chronic, continual stressors by bolstering resiliency It can help nurses develop coping skills to deal the stressors around end-of-life and bereavement care It can help develop resourcefulness and resiliency skills by changing the way one views stressors (eg, overwhelming and hopeless to something that is coped with and learned from)	There are many recommended training programs on CBT An example of one CBT technique: When one feels angry or stressed, stop and think: What are my thoughts? Are these helping me handle the situation or not? What thoughts could I be thinking instead?
Positive thinking/positive psychology	May help develop optimism and cognitive flexibility	Keep a log of thoughts for 1 wk to identify any negative thinking patterns (eg, blaming or perfection) Practice taking these negative thoughts and replace them with reasonable alternatives
Gratitude practice	Creates a greater sense of well-being and may help lower symptoms of depression	Write down 3–5 things that one is grateful for daily Do this for 30 d If this practice is helpful after 30 d, continue the practice Another suggestion is to express sincere appreciation for others on a regular basis
Daily release ritual	Rituals are symbolic activities that can relieve anxiety, provide comfort, meaning, and support when	Begin by reviewing the day and any challenging situations faced Next, acknowledge that it is harmful to carry around

(continued on next page)

Table 2
(continued)

Type	Benefit	Suggestions and Examples
	dealing with uncertainties, such as those faced at the end of life	these emotions from the day Then, practice letting these emotions go This ritual can be done while listening to music on the drive home or before sleep, while changing clothes after work, while meditating or praying, while bathing or showering Visualizing washing away the day's concerns or visualizing these concerns going down the drain or getting further and further away from you
Sacred pause ritual	May help lower distress and burnout	An ICU team member thanks and acknowledges the efforts of the team and the patient's family and honors the life of the patient who just died Then the team observes a 1-min pause
Remembrance	Practice where the team can safely remember patients and acknowledge emotions they may be experiencing	Four main components discussed during rounds once a week: 1. Acknowledge the deaths of recent patients 2. Reflect on the psychological and/or spiritual impact these deaths may have had on the team 3. Discuss bereavement risk for families 4. Model self-care strategies to help team members cope
Humor and laughter therapy	Humor and laughter can increase immune function, relax muscles, reduce stress, and improve mood Humor and laughter can increase energy levels, decrease stress, decrease the burden of grief, and improve well-being	Leaving humorous books in the break room Posting jokes on the bulletin board Use humor carefully to ensure that it is not disrespectful or offensive
Education: In-services on grief ELNEC/end-of-life tool kits	Promotes comfort and competence in providing end-of-life care	Periodic staff education programs on end-of-life and bereavement care, offering continuing education credits for incentive Hold in-services on grief

Counseling	Help resolve issues and help deal with grief, stress, and other distressing emotions	Provide access to an employee assistance program, a counsellor, or a psychologist to support nurses dealing with patient deaths
Other techniques	Soothing outlets that may help provide an emotional release	Watch a movie that stimulates crying Listen to music Expressive writing or journaling Creating (eg, arts, crafts, knitting) Practice self-compassion (being kind to oneself) Enjoying a hot bath "to wash away the day" Pet therapy Aromatherapy Massage therapy Gardening (eg, plant "new" life) Cleaning ("clean away the day")

Abbreviations: CBT, cognitive behavioral therapy; ELNEC, End-of-Life Nursing Education Consortium; ICU, intensive care unit.
Data from Refs. [6,7,14,19,23,25,28,36-38,40-46]

Table 3
Personal and professional relationship self-care techniques

Type	Benefit	Suggestions and Examples
Support from family and friends	The emotionally demanding work of critical care makes a strong support system essential Finding those able to listen and support is crucial	Educate significant others and friends about work stresses and ways they can offer meaningful support Be alert to warning signals, such as overextending, not setting limits, and handling conflicts by blaming or personalizing Set healthy limits in personal and professional relationships Handle conflict directly with the person involved and handle difficult issues as soon as possible
Formal and informal support from colleagues: Support groups Debriefing Sharing narratives and stories	Helpful in preventing burnout and compassion fatigue These techniques can assist in managing emotions, maintaining confidence and self-esteem, normalizing experiences, and developing new resources and coping methods	Regularly schedule formal debriefing sessions after a patient's death Seek out informal debriefing with trusted colleagues Have peer support groups available if possible Check-in with team members on how they are feeling, remind each other of the importance of self-care

Data from Refs.[7,8,23,28,36]

calmness, serenity, and hope.[28] For example, Kathy could discover her interest in photography. She could start making collages with her photographs and find this to be a relaxing and renewing activity. **Box 4** lists techniques that the critical care nurse can use to develop a stronger spiritual connection and renewal and develop a sense of perspective and meaning that goes beyond the day-to-day life.[23,25,28]

AUTHENTIC LEADERSHIP AND THE IMPORTANCE TO SELF-CARE

In addition to the prior areas we discussed, having a healthy work environment, with authentic leaders, is just as crucial to the nurses' health and well-being. This type of work environment has been associated with lower risk of moral distress, burnout, and compassion fatigue in critical care nurses.[48,49] In this type of environment, leaders focus on the health and well-being of the individual nurse and on the whole system. Authentic nurse leaders are mindful, open, honest, neutral, accountable, and positive.[50] They are skilled at creating environments where nurses flourish.[50] These leaders create environments where nurses feel supported and feel like they can contribute to meaningful work.[50] This type of leadership promotes and encourages self-care in the workplace[25]; in essence these leaders normalize self-care.[8]

For example, Kathy's nurse manager sensed that the staff were suffering from low morale after caring for so many dying patients over the last month. The manager discussed with the nursing staff systems that would best support them. Using a collaborative process, the nurse manager and the nurses decide that after any patient death, the primary nurse needs to be provided with additional time to practice self-care. The nurse would be encouraged to take a break and perform any activity that helps clear the mind before resuming their regular duties. **Box 5** provides self-care suggestions that critical care nurse leaders can initiate to create healthy work environments around end-of-life and bereavement care.[5,7,8,14,20,23,28,36,50,51]

SUMMARY

Providing end-of-life and bereavement care is a rewarding experience but can also lead to cumulative grief, compassion fatigue, and burnout. Critical care nurses can protect their health and well-being through developing and practicing self-care techniques that focus on enhancing their physical, emotional, personal and professional relationships, and spiritual health. Critical care leadership is also integral in supporting

---

Box 4
Spiritual self-care techniques

- Meditation and reflection
- Reading prayer, scripture, or spiritual books
- Attending religious or spiritual services
- Participating in nature activities (eg, hiking, mindful walking)
- Practicing forgiveness
- Practicing gratitude
- Practicing photography and creating collages
- Involvement in other aspects of life (eg, gathering with friends and family)

Data from Refs.[23,25,28]

Box 5
Authentic leadership activities to improve self-care

- Offer regular in-services on self-care
- Promote the importance of self-care to staff on a regular basis
- Reward self-care behaviors (eg, a nurse who stays home to get well rather than coming into work sick)
- Create spaces where nurses can get away from the stressors at work and process their emotions
- Ensure nurses receive regular breaks throughout the shift
- Ensure nurses take regular vacations throughout the year
- Offer yearly retreats to refresh and regroup as a team
- Manage workload, ensure that it is not excessive
- Provide adequate staffing
- Consider mentoring junior nurses with an experienced nurse during challenging end-of-life situations
- Manage the caseload for a nurse following the death of a patient by allowing the nurse to focus their care on the deceased and their family

Data from Refs.[5,7,8,14,20,23,28,36,50,51]

---

this type of care to maintain a healthy workforce. By integrating some of these techniques Kathy improved awareness of her self-care needs and implemented some techniques, such as regularly meeting a coworker for coffee every week. Recently, she found a book in the break room and was inspired by the following quote: "For someone to develop genuine compassion toward others, first he or she must have a basis on which to cultivate compassion, and that basis is the ability to connect to one's own feelings and to care for one's own welfare. . . Caring for others requires caring for oneself."[52(p125)]

She placed it on bulletin board to remind herself and other colleagues the importance of caring for themselves. Critical care nurses are experts in providing compassionate care to patients and their families at their most vulnerable times in life. The essence of self-care is turning that compassion inward, so that nurses' own wells are full and they are able to continuing giving to others.

DISCLOSURE

The authors have nothing to disclose.

REFERENCES

1. Efstathiou N, Walker W, Metcalfe A, et al. The state of bereavement support in adult intensive care: a systematic review and narrative synthesis. J Crit Care 2019;50:177–87.

2. Powazki R, Walsh D, Cothren B, et al. The care of the actively dying in an academic medical center: a survey of registered nurses' professional capability and comfort. Am J Hosp Palliat Care 2014;31(6):619–27.

3. Shariff A, Olson J, Salas AS, et al. Nurses' experiences of providing care to bereaved families who experience unexpected death in intensive care units: a narrative overview. Can J Crit Care Nurs 2017;28(1):21–9.

4. McAdam JL, Erikson A. Bereavement services offered in adult intensive care units in the United States. Am J Crit Care 2016;25(2):110–7.

5. Broden EG, Uveges MK. Applications of grief and bereavement theory for critical care nurses. AACN Adv Crit Care 2018;29(3):354–9.

6. Kapoor S, Morgan CK, Siddique MA, et al. "Sacred pause" in the ICU: evaluation of a ritual and intervention to lower distress and burnout. Am J Hosp Palliat Care 2018;35(10):1337–41.

7. Kisorio LC, Langley GC. Intensive care nurses' experiences of end-of-life care. Intensive Crit Care Nurs 2016;33:30–8.

8. Mills J, Wand T, Fraser JA. Exploring the meaning and practice of self-care among palliative care nurses and doctors: a qualitative study. BMC Palliat Care 2018;17(1):63.

9. Wolf AT, White KR, Epstein EG, et al. Palliative care and moral distress: an institutional survey of critical care nurses. Crit Care Nurse 2019;39(5):38–49.

10. Luckett A. End-of-life care guidelines and care plans in the intensive care unit. Br J Nurs 2017;26(5):287–93.

11. Davidson JE, Aslakson RA, Long AC, et al. Guidelines for family-centered care in the neonatal, pediatric, and adult ICU. Crit Care Med 2017;45(1):103–28.

12. Ahluwalia SC, Chen C, Raaen L, et al. A systematic review in support of the national consensus project clinical practice guidelines for quality palliative care, fourth edition. J Pain Symptom Manage 2018;56(6):831–70.

13. Endacott R, Boyer C, Benbenishty J, et al. Perceptions of a good death: a qualitative study in intensive care units in England and Israel. Intensive Crit Care Nurs 2016;36:8–16.

14. Funk LM, Peters S, Roger KS. The emotional labor of personal grief in palliative care: balancing caring and professional identities. Qual Health Res 2017; 27(14):2211–21.

15. Naidoo V, Sibiya M. Experiences of critical care nurses of death and dying in an intensive care unit: a phenomenological study. J Nurs Care 2014;3(179):1–4. https://doi.org/10.4172/2167-1168.1000179.

16. Shorter M, Stayt LC. Critical care nurses' experiences of grief in an adult intensive care unit. J Adv Nurs 2010;66(1):159–67.

17. Boyle DA. Countering compassion fatigue: a requisite nursing agenda. Online J Issues Nurs 2011;16(1):2.

18. Mealer M, Conrad D, Evans J, et al. Feasibility and acceptability of a resilience training program for intensive care unit nurses. Am J Crit Care 2014;23(6): e97–105.

19. Pospos S, Young IT, Downs N, et al. Web-based tools and mobile applications to mitigate burnout, depression, and suicidality among healthcare students and professionals: a systematic review. Acad Psychiatry 2018;42(1):109–20.

20. van Mol MM, Kompanje EJ, Benoit DD, et al. The prevalence of compassion fatigue and burnout among healthcare professionals in intensive care units: a systematic review. PLoS One 2015;10(8):1–22, e0136955.

21. Chuang CH, Tseng PC, Lin CY, et al. Burnout in the intensive care unit professionals: a systematic review. Medicine (Baltimore) 2016;95(50):e5629.

22. Mills J, Wand T, Fraser JA. On self-compassion and self-care in nursing: selfish or essential for compassionate care? Int J Nurs Stud 2015;52(4):791–3.

23. Butler LD, Mercer KA, McClain-Meeder K, et al. Six domains of self-care: attending to the whole person. J Hum Behav Soc Environ 2019;29(1):107–24.

24. Davies N. A crash course in grief. Nurs Stand 2015;30(5):72.

25. Crane PJ, Ward SF. Self-healing and self-care for nurses. AORN J 2016;104(5): 386–400.

26. Caffrey PM. A gentle reminder to make time for yourself. Available at: https://www.calvaryhospital.org/self-care-for-palliative-care-professionals/. Accessed October 7, 2019.

27. Dyrbye LN, Johnson PO, Johnson LM, et al. Efficacy of the well-being index to identify distress and well-being in U.S. nurses. Nurs Res 2018;67(6):447–55.

28. Smit C. Making self-care a priority. Whitireia Nursing & Health Journal 2017;24: 29–35.

29. Yaribeygi H, Panahi Y, Sahraei H, et al. The impact of stress on body function: a review. EXCLI J 2017;16:1057–72.

30. Blum CA. Practicing self-care for nurses: a nursing program initiative. Online J Issues Nurs 2014;19(3):3.

31. CDC. How much sleep do I need?. 2017. Available at: https://www.cdc.gov/sleep/about_sleep/how_much_sleep.html. Accessed October 8, 2019.

32. CDC. Physical activity basics. 2019. Available at: https://www.cdc.gov/physicalactivity/basics/. Accessed October 8, 2019.

33. Epel ES, Crosswell AD, Mayer SE, et al. More than a feeling: a unified view of stress measurement for population science. Front Neuroendocrinol 2018;49: 146–69.

34. Duarte J, Pinto-Gouveia J. Effectiveness of a mindfulness-based intervention on oncology nurses' burnout and compassion fatigue symptoms: a non-randomized study. Int J Nurs Stud 2016;64:98–107.

35. Scott E. Reduce stress and improve your life with positive self talk. 2019. Available at: https://www.verywellmind.com/how-to-use-positive-self-talk-for-stress-relief-3144816. Accessed October 24, 2019.

36. Bajer L. Personal reflection: death brokering for critical care nurses. Dimens Crit Care Nurs 2012;31(5):287–9.

37. Gauthier T, Meyer RM, Grefe D, et al. An on-the-job mindfulness-based intervention for pediatric ICU nurses: a pilot. J Pediatr Nurs 2015;30(2):402–9.

38. Halm M. The role of mindfulness in enhancing self-care for nurses. Am J Crit Care 2017;26(4):344–8.

39. Harbaugh CN, Vasey MW. When do people benefit from gratitude practice? J Posit Psychol 2014;9(6):535–46.

40. Montross-Thomas LP, Scheiber C, Meier EA, et al. Personally meaningful rituals: a way to increase compassion and decrease burnout among hospice staff and volunteers. J Palliat Med 2016;19(10):1043–50.

41. Morris SE, Kearns JP, Moment A, et al. "Remembrance": a self-care tool for clinicians. J Palliat Med 2019;22(3):316–8.

42. Nunes IR, Jose H, Capelas ML. Grieving with humor. Holist Nurs Pract 2018; 32(2):98–106.

43. Yim J. Therapeutic benefits of laughter in mental health: a theoretical review. Tohoku J Exp Med 2016;239(3):243–9.

44. Steinberg BA, Klatt M, Duchemin AM. Feasibility of a mindfulness-based intervention for surgical intensive care unit personnel. Am J Crit Care 2016; 26(1):10–8.

45. Ferrell B, Malloy P, Virani R. The end of life nursing education nursing consortium project. Ann Palliat Med 2015;4(2):61–9.

46. Eberth J, Sedlmeier P. The effects of mindfulness meditation: a meta-analysis. Mindfulness 2012;3:174–89.

47. Meller N, Parker D, Hatcher D, et al. Grief experiences of nurses after the death of an adult patient in an acute hospital setting: an integrative review of literature. Collegian 2019;26:302–10.

48. Hickey PA. A vision for excellence by design. Am J Crit Care 2019;28(4):247–54.

49. Kowalski MO, Basile C, Bersick E, et al. What do nurses need to practice effectively in the hospital environment? An integrative review with implications for nurse leaders. Worldviews Evid Based Nurs 2020;17(1):60–70.

50. Ward SF, Haase B. Conscious leadership. AORN J 2016;104(5):433.e1-9.

51. Endacott R. 'I cried too' - allowing ICU nurses to grieve when patients die. Intensive Crit Care Nurs 2019;52:1–2.

52. Lama D. Transforming the mind: teachings on generating compassion. Hammersmith (London): Thorsons; 2003.

Integrative Health and Wellness Assessment Tool

Deborah McElligott, DNP, ANP-BC, AHN-BC, HWNC-BC, CDE[a,b,c,*],
Joanne Turnier, DNP, RN, ACNS-BC, HN-BC, HWNC-BC[d,e,1]

KEYWORDS

- Integrative assessment • Burnout • Health and wellness coaching • Self-care
- Critical care nurses • Theory of Integrative Nurse Coaching

KEY POINTS

- Integrative self-assessment is a first step in supporting goals and action steps to decrease burnout and enhance well-being in critical care nurses.
- The Theory of Integrative Nurse Coaching supports self-care in critical care nurses as an individual journey or a unit-based process.
- The IHWA tool can be integrated into coaching sessions for diverse populations in any setting.

INTRODUCTION

The purpose of this article is to discuss the background and use of the Integrative Health and Wellness Assessment (IHWA)[1] Tool as it relates to critical care nursing. Although the foundation of nursing is grounded in holistic nursing theory and practice, the nature of the critical care environment often pulls the nurse into a task-oriented model. In an effort to address the serious life-sustaining requirements of the patient, document appropriately in the electronic record, and meet institutional mandates, critical care nurses may lose their focus on the whole patient. This can lead to fragmentation in care, discontentment, job dissatisfaction, burnout, and loss of meaning in their nursing practice.

[a] Center for Wellness & Integrative Medicine, Katz Institute for Women's Health, Northwell Health, Roslyn, NY, USA; [b] International Nurse Coach Association, North Miami, FL, USA; [c] Donald and Barbara Zucker School of Medicine at Hofstra/Northwell, Uniondale, NY, USA; [d] International Nurse Coach Association; [e] Center for Wellness and Integrative Medicine, Roslyn, NY, USA
[1] Present address: Dreamworks Court, Fort Solonga, NY 11768.
* Corresponding author. PO Box 551, Point Lookout, NY 11569.
E-mail address: hnpcoach@gmail.com

Crit Care Nurs Clin N Am 32 (2020) 439–450
https://doi.org/10.1016/j.cnc.2020.05.006
0899-5885/20/© 2020 Elsevier Inc. All rights reserved.

In 2014 the Institute for Healthcare Improvement introduced a framework known as the Triple Aim, a 3-dimensional approach to optimizing health system performance.[2] The Triple Aim includes improving the patient experience, the health of populations, and reducing per capita costs of health care. As the Triple Aim shifted to the Quadruple Aim, and added the fourth dimension "improving the work life of health care clinicians and staff," a focus on health care workers surfaced. Quality of care, patient safety, outcomes, and cost containment are significantly linked to the well-being of the nurse and to other health care professionals.

Health professionals and the general population are increasingly affected by chronic disease and lifestyle choices. To address this challenge, the nurse coach role was developed, supported by both nursing and change theories.[3] This role spans the spectrum of nursing, incorporating coaching skills in all areas of nursing, including critical care. In this role, an integrative assessment is essential. Instruments such as the IHWA serve as a fundamental assessment enabling the nurse coach and critical care nurses to expand their (self) awareness through reflection and improve their respective self-care.

Therefore, this article discusses the role of integrative health, holistic nursing, nurse coaching, and the need for the critical care nurse to implement sustainable self-care strategies. The IHWA facilitates the preceding process and is highlighted throughout this article.

INTEGRATIVE HEALTH

As the National Center for Complementary and Alternative Medicine changed their name to the National Center for Complementary and Integrative Health in 2016, they reflected the changing views of the world and the increased use of Integrative approaches, theories and concepts.[4] Therapies including but not limited to yoga, massage, meditation, acupuncture, reflexology, Tai Chi, energy therapies, and natural supplements have dramatically increased in use among both clients and health care practitioners.[5] With this name change, the term Integrative Health began to appear in many different settings, with various definitions.

Wayne Jonas, MD, describes Integrative Health as a combination of the best of conventional medical care, complementary and alternative care, and a large focus on self-care.[6] Integrative health care may be defined as a focus on whole person/whole systems care grounded in prevention and relationships and delivered by interprofessional teams that include conventional and complementary/alternative therapies.[7]

Essential to the delivery of care via an integrative approach, is the integrative assessment. Similar to the definition, there are many forms or recommendations for an integrative assessment with most focusing on whole person assessment and the concept of healing. The whole person concept recognizes that the person is more than their disease, age, or culture; a unique individual experiencing a disease process who is surrounded by and constantly interacting with their internal and external environment. This environment encompasses the health care team, family, physical environment, and community. The concept of healing as opposed to a focus on curing gives new meaning to the critical care nurse who may not be able to cure a patient of his or her disease but can certainly participate in the healing process on some level, even as the patient is dying.

CRITICAL CARE NURSING

Critical care nurses are exposed to intense situations that involve the caring for patients and families who are experiencing serious physical, psychological, and social problems.[8] The high levels of burnout in critical care nursing are attributed to the stressful work environment of the intensive care unit (ICU) caused by high patient morbidity and mortality, challenging daily work routines, and regular encounters with traumatic events and ethical issues.[9] Additional conflicts arise if the nurses' personal values are in conflict with the values of the health care team or patient and the patient's family. These stressful interactions place critical care nurses at great risk for posttraumatic stress disorder, alcohol abuse, and suicidal thoughts.[9] Burnout has serious implications for nurses, patients, and organizational health care and is linked to a reduction in quality of care, lower patient satisfaction, and increased numbers of medical errors, higher rates of health care–associated infections, and higher 30-day patient mortality rates.[9]

Although it is important to focus on measures that address stressful ICU environments, it is also important for critical care nurses to take the time to carefully assess all aspects of self, influencing the personal perceptions of stress. In doing so, nurses may find a way to reconnect with inner wisdom and incorporate meaningful self-care strategies to promote healing and a sense of well-being. By taking responsibility to make optimal life choices, critical care nurses will become better positioned to create healthier patterns that promote healing and enhance personal resilience, and model that behavior for patients.

The literature suggests that self-care workshops, stress reduction programs, nurse coaching, mindfulness meditation, changes in workload scheduling, exercise, and organizational and individual accountability significantly reduce the effects of burnout.[10,11] Significant improvement in health-promoting behaviors of nurses has been noted when a holistic approach was used at the unit level with a program that focused on unit goals and coaching techniques.[12]

This issue of self-care for nurses has been a focus of the American Nurses Association, for years and highlighted in the 2017 Healthy Nurse Healthy Nation efforts.[13] Numerous nurses and institutions throughout the country have supported the national call for all nurses to model the healthy behaviors they ask their patients to embrace. Whitehead[14] described a disparity between nursing expert opinions on health promotion and the actual translation into practice by bedside nurses. Despite the findings in the literature, and the support of national organizations, a gap between knowing the importance of self-care and actually implementing a successful sustainable self-care plan continues to exist within the nursing profession.

HOLISTIC NURSING

For decades the American Holistic Nurses Association has titled one core value as Self-Care of the nurse, highlighting the importance of whole person caring and linking the health of the nurse to the outcomes of patient care.[15] Nursing is one of the few professions that has taken the lead in the holistic, integrative approach to well-being and healing for all people. Although integrative terminology may not always be used, a holistic approach began with the work of Nightingale,[16] who identified the integral nature of the person-environment system, which is evident in nursing practice today. This approach is supported by the work of numerous nursing theorists and their theories including, but not limited to, Watson (Caring Science)[17] and Dossey (Integral theory).[18] Each of those grand theories support the importance of whole-person assessment, the therapeutic healing environment, and the caring presence of the nurse. However, nursing grand theories that support caring and self-care may be difficult to implement at the bedside, especially in the critical care unit.

THE THEORY OF INTEGRATIVE NURSE COACHING

The mid-range Theory of Integrative Nurse Coaching (TINC),[19] developed to guide the practice of nurse coaches, encompasses many holistic nursing theories and provides support for lifestyle changes and well-being both for the nurse and the client. The theory is composed of concepts such as healing, the metaparadigm in nursing, patterns of knowing, and 5 components (**Fig. 1**).

Although TINC includes 5 components, this article addresses Component 1, Self-development, where one takes responsibility for their learning and growth. Self-development is paramount to one's nursing career and aligns with one's own healing journey and transformation to wholeness.[20] The component of self-development includes various processes, in a continuous integral process.

- *Self-reflection* is turning inward for self-examination of thoughts, values, beliefs, experiences, and inner wisdom.[21] It is the continuous thread in self-development, as it integrates the heart with the critically thinking mind throughout

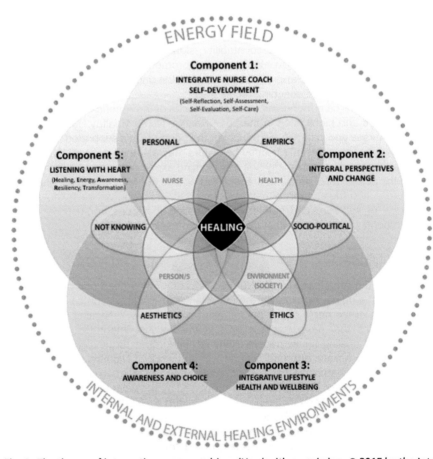

Fig. 1. The theory of integrative nurse coaching. (Used with permission. © 2015 by the International Nurse Coach Association. www.inursecoach.com.)

self-assessment, self-evaluation, and self-care.[22] Reflection supports new relationships, as critical care nurses form deeper relationships and learn to "be with" both themselves and their patients.[22] A daily practice of self-reflection (eg, mindfulness, meditation, imagery, breath awareness) enables nurses to harness these skills in the heat of the unit, in the face of ambiguity, and retrieve a sense of clarity and therapeutic presence.

- *Self-assessment* includes both formal and informal assessments, conventional medical and nursing assessments, as well as integrative assessments, thus embracing integrative health.
- *Self-evaluation* explores our understanding of experiences and behaviors. It may often occur as we evaluate goal achievement.
- *Self-care* is the process of engaging in health-related activities to enhance balance and well-being. Principles of self-care include a positive self-image, positive attitude, self-discipline and integration of body-mind-spirit.[21]

This framework for practice in the nurse's own self-development mirrors the coaching structure that enhances the care of their patients and the patients' self-development. The nurse, through the therapeutic relationships, assists the client via a discovery model to identify a first step on his or her path to well-being. Building on strengths, inner wisdom, values and past success, the nurse in a coaching role assists patients in defining their hope, and determining where they need to begin in the change process, as they identify goals and action plans. This structure supports patient-centered care and the magnet standards institutions seek to uphold.

INTEGRATIVE HEALTH AND WELLNESS ASSESSMENT

The IHWA[23] may be the first step in supporting the self-development of the critical care nurses, as it helps them to reflect on their wellness status via 8 dimensions of wellness, introducing them to an integrative self-assessment. The tool was developed in 2011 as a 132-question Likert scale tool, based on more than 30 years of integrative, integral, and holistic nursing clinical practice, education, and research to address the dimensions of wellness as defined by the TINC (see **Fig. 1**). These dimensions are also included in a shorter form (36 questions) that was later developed to support the self-assessment and self-reflection needs of nurses, especially in a time-limited coaching practice.[23]

The tool fosters self-assessment through a reflective process, but may also be used as an outcome measurement, as baseline scores may be compared before and after lifestyle changes. Total scores on the 36-item, 5-point Likert scale IHWA may range from 36 to 180. Psychometric testing of the short form revealed an overall Cronbach alpha of 0.88; Kaiser-Meyer-Olkin value of 0.520, and the Bartlett test of sphericity was significant. Thus the short form is valid as an overall measure of wellness, whereas further testing is recommended to improve subscales.[23]

DIMENSIONS OF THE INTEGRATIVE HEALTH AND WELLNESS ASSESSMENT

The IHWA offers an integrative approach to assessment through 8 components of wellness: (1) Life Balance and Satisfaction, (2) Relationships, (3) Spiritual, (4) Mental, (5) Emotional, (6) Physical (Nutrition, Exercise, Weight Management), and (8) Health Responsibility (**Fig. 2**).[23]

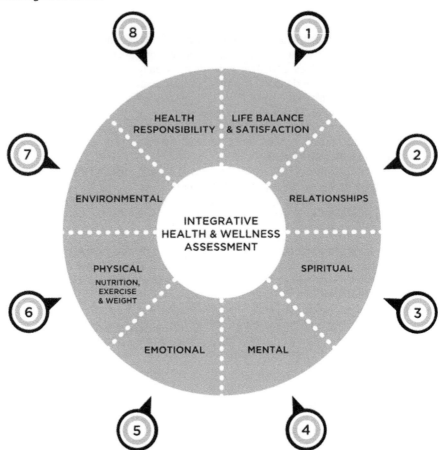

Fig. 2. Integrative Health and Wellness Assessment wheel. (Copyright © 2015. Used with permission. International Nurse Coach Association. www.inursecoach.com.)

- Assessment of *Life Balance and Satisfaction* includes a recognition and celebration of joys, strengths, and positive aspects of life. One's awareness of conscious choices and the unconscious influences are raised.
- *Relationships* are assessed through self-reflection, to identify whether they are cohesive or disharmonious, superficial or deeply connected.
- *Spiritual* assessment often involves a sense of connection with something greater than ourselves and is aligned to our meaning and purpose.
- *Mental* assessment involves review of one's belief systems, values, and conflicts.
- *Emotional* assessment includes the acknowledgment of our full range of feelings (including love, joy, compassion, fear, anger, guilt, forgiveness) and the way we express them.
- *Physical* assessment involves evaluation of behaviors surrounding nutrition, weight, and physical activity.
- *Health Responsibility* includes complying with annual screening recommendations, identifying and addressing symptoms and risk factors.
- *Environmental* assessment includes the impact of our internal and external environment on our health and well-being.

THE INTEGRATIVE HEALTH AND WELLNESS ASSESSMENT AND CHANGE THEORY

Praxis describes the translation of theory into a practice setting. In this particular case the self-development component of Dossey, Luck and Schaub's mid-range Theory of Integrative Nurse Coaching can be seamlessly integrated into the lives of critical care nurses. The utilization of the IHWA offers critical care nurses the opportunity to assess personal challenges and discover new behaviors that enhance their ability to self-assess, reflect, and explore. This empowers them to implement self-care strategies that promote healing and a sense of well-being. Although the IHWA serves as an initial step in the critical care nurse's ability to self-assess, it is important to realize that without intervention, lasting change will not be achievable or sustainable. Although behavioral change may appear simple, it is important for critical care nurses to understand the fundamental reasons for their behavior, barriers to change, and internal and external motivations that cause either conflict or promote a positive outcome.

The Transtheoretical Model of Behavioral Change highlights the stages of change that gauge readiness.[24] Each stage is described as follows and supports specific coaching actions.

- The "Pre-contemplative" stage describes a person's lack of interest in changing behavior, which may result from past failures or unsuccessful attempts to change.
- During the "Contemplative" stage of the model, the pros and cons and the benefits of change are considered. Individuals are more likely to initiate behavioral changes when they are dissatisfied with their current situation. Once ambivalent feelings are resolved, options and intention to adopt healthier behavior is further considered.
- During the "Preparing for Action" stage, individuals are aware of their personal challenges and barriers and have clear intention to implement behavioral changes.
- In the "Taking Action" phase, new behaviors are identified and consistently integrated. The potential for relapses and returning to old behaviors may occur during this stage so it is important to illicit unit and or community support.
- The "Maintenance" stage happens when new behaviors become habits and are automatically mastered. During this phase, it is vital to celebrate accomplishments and avoid relapses.[24]

To achieve lasting behavioral change, it is vital that organizations support critical care practice settings and encourage critical care nurses to implement self-care practices on a unit level. For critical care nurses, even those who use a holistic approach to patient care, completion of the IHWA tool often provides unexpected insights, and shifts the focus beyond the body, mind, and spirit to include other dimensions. Although reflection and self-assessment may identify desires for change, implementing change as an individual can be challenging. Forming partnerships with nurses who are coaches is a logical next step and one way to effect desired change via an integrative model.

Just as nursing practice is guided by the nursing process, the nurse coaching process guides interactions for nurse coaches.[3] The case study in **Table 1** identifies the use of the IHWA in a coaching session between an ICU nurse and a nurse coach.

The 8 components of the IHWA may also be used in a group coaching setting such as a focus on workplace wellness. Unit staff could complete the IHWA and then discuss results in a safe setting and determine goals that would enhance the health and well-being of all. Strategies that may be used for either individual or group settings are included in **Table 2**.

Table 1
Using the Integrative Health and Wellness Assessment (IHWA) in a coaching session

Sue's Story	Nurse Coaching Process (6 Steps)
Referral process: Registered nurse (RN) to Nurse Coach (NC) Sue, a 48-year-old ICU RN seeks health and wellness coaching to improve her pre-diabetes (HgA1c 6.0; fasting blood sugar of 120). She gained 15 pounds over the past 2 years, and had family history of diabetes.	*The goal of nurse coaching is to partner with patients who have the desire and readiness to make changes. Change is a process involving self-assessment, goals, action plans, and self-evaluation*
The NC explains the coaching process, and Sue describes her reason for coming to the session. The NC listens to her story and explores her hopes, unique challenges, strengths, and skills. Sue fears a diagnosis of diabetes due to her family history. She highlights her recent laboratory results, busy work schedule, and sugary snacking habits to keep alert during the night shift. Sue also states that she has no time or energy to exercise. She lives alone, often orders "take out" and is annoyed with her weight gain, because she "knows what to do."	1. *Establishing Relationship and Identifying Readiness for Change (Assessment):* The NC prepares for the session by centering and then partners with the patient to identify strengths, desired change, and readiness for change. *The NC allows the patient's story to unfold; the patient is in control of the session, which increases self-efficacy and self-confidence. Skills such as SMART Goals, Motivational Interviewing, Appreciative Inquiry, and Brief Action Planning are used.*
Sue agrees to be guided through a breath awareness practice.	The NC guides Sue into a focused breath awareness to assist with relaxation.
Sue is given an IHWA to assist with self-assessment and identify areas of strengths and challenges. She identifies difficulty with the components of life balance and satisfaction, mental, spiritual, physical and emotional, with concerns that they are impacting both her job performance and overall health. She loves her work in the intensive care unit (ICU), and reports difficulty with her recent shift change and short staffing. She has difficulty sleeping, irregular eating patterns, and an increased number of sick days due to fatigue. Sue also describes a typical workday and perceived barriers to health.	2. *Identifying Opportunities, Issues, and Concerns (Diagnosis):* The NC partners with the patient to identify opportunities and issues related to growth, overall health, wholeness, and well-being. Opportunities for celebrating well-being are explored; acknowledgment promotes and reinforces previous successes and serves to enhance further achievements. *There is no need to establish a diagnosis. The patient chooses the session topic and sets the pace. The NC holds a therapeutic presence to Sue's story and avoids the desire to "fix" as each patient is the expert on what currently works and what does not work.*
Sue is overwhelmed with over all the "things" she needs to do to be healthy and asks the NC where to begin. The NC summarizes the information she provided and holds the silence until Sue responds. Sue was allowed to determine the direction of the coaching conversation around her areas of interest. The NC asked, "What is one health-related behavior you would like to change within the next week?" Sue identifies stress and hoped to incorporate the breath awareness into her	3. *Establishing Patient-Centered Goals (Outcomes Identification): Allowing clients to set the pace, summarizing what was said and holding space supports reflection. This may increase the patient's motivation and invite a possible change. The Brief Action Plan (BAP) is often used to assist a patient to implement one change. It involves 3 questions regarding the desired change, confidence in ability to carry out the plan, (her confidence was a 7/10) and a check-in to review how the*

(continued on next page)

Table 1	
(continued)	
Sue's Story	**Nurse Coaching Process (6 Steps)**
daily life. She shared that she was confident that she could use this technique 5/7 d a week in the morning for 5 min each day. She asked for more resources for self-care.	plan is going. If a confidence level is <7, it is recommended that the plan be revised until confidence is >7. The NC gave Sue the link to the AHNA Self-care toolkit.[25]
Sue sought 12 coaching sessions to assist her in incorporating lifestyle changes with an initial focus on stress management.	4. Creating the Structure of the Coaching Interaction (Planning): The NC and Sue developed an agreement for weekly sessions, discussing the timing and length of sessions.
Completion of first session: Sue remarked that she felt relief with this 1 goal, as initially there were many areas that she felt needed attention. She agreed to log her thoughts and activities around food, stress, and activity for 5 d. Her confidence level for being able to log these activities was 8/10.	5. Empowering and Motivating Patients to Reach Goals (Implementation): The NC uses deep listening, and skillful questioning during the coaching interaction. In partnership with the patient, the NC co-creates an environment that allows the client to prioritize, design action plans, and set goals.
Sue worked with the NC for 12 weekly sessions over 3 mo. Each week, progress and challenges were reviewed and Sue reset SMART Goals. Her personal story unfolded and the recognition of her strengths helped to create new dreams. In subsequent sessions Sue focused on increasing activity and choosing healthy foods.	The NC supported Sue's new awareness and choices at each session, Sue saw new possibilities, creating her vision for health. She had a greater understanding, meaning, and insight around personal lifestyle choices, which she noticed had a positive effect on her work environment with both her peers and patients.
Patient Summary. Sue reported: "I felt listened to and supported by my NC." "I recognize my strengths and resiliency to better manage my life challenges." "I lost 10 pounds, improved my energy, sleep, and self-image." "Work is different now and I am more focused with less fatigue after the shift." "My A1C went from 6 to 5.6." "I use relaxation techniques during my shift to help me cope with ICU stressors."	6. Assisting Patient to Determine the Extent to which Goals were Achieved (Evaluation): Evaluation of coaching is done primarily by the patient, based on their perception of success and achievement of created goals. Sue's story represents the power of integrative assessment and coaching. Although she focused on "parts" as reflected in the IHWA, she recognized that a change in one area impacts many other areas of wellness.

Table 2
Integrative health and wellness components

Wellness Component	Self-Reflection	Self-Care Strategy	Critical Care Unit Strategy
Emotional	Do I recognize my own feelings and emotions?	Daily journal: consider gratitude journal on a daily basis for 21 days	How can the unit staff respond instead of react? Set a 5-min unit daily meditation or reflection
Mental	Do I have compassion for myself as I set my personal goals?	Assess readiness to change and set a SMART goal	Create a safe space for reflection
Spiritual	Do I find meaning, value and purpose in my nursing practice?	Begin a daily contemplative practice for at least 10 min/d	How does our work reflect our mission and vision-does it align with our values
Physical	How does my activity and nutrition support my health?	Consider a food and activity journal for at least 1 wk	Can we ensure each of us have a break for meals and access to healthy food?
Environmental	Do I have a healthy nontoxic environment?	What products do I use on my body and what chemicals are in my food?	What environmental toxins are in our workplace and how can we change them (eg, products, sound, relationships)
Health responsibility	Do I pay attention to my physical well-being and address symptoms as they arise?	Do I follow recommendations for healthy living?	How does our unit foster our health?
Relationships	Do I have satisfying relationships with myself, my family, and others?	Am I compassionate and nonjudgmental with myself and others?	How do our work relationships support our healing?
Life balance and satisfaction	Do I have balance among work, family friends, and self-care?	How do my choices enhance my potential?	What was the best day we had in the past month at work? How do we create more of those days?

SUMMARY

The role of the critical care nurse continues to evolve in complexity and demand, with the cost of replacing critical care nurses ever rising. Challenges exist to sustain the health and well-being of these nurses and to support their development of self-care skills to sustain the meaning and joy in their nursing practice. A daily self-reflective practice is a cornerstone of the self-development and cannot be underemphasized. Self-assessment and self-care are priorities for both the nurse as an individual, the unit as a team, and the care of the patients and families they serve. The TINC, with a core focus on healing, and the IHWA, as structure for self-assessment, combined with coaching skills, supports the development of self-care plans that include realistic and attainable goals.

As critical care nurses embrace integrative approaches to their health and well-being, including their own integrative self-assessment, focused on self-care, they embrace the meaning and begin to integrate the principles of Healthy Nurse Healthy Nation into their daily lives. Through these new learned behaviors, nurses pave an optimistic path for the future of the nursing profession and the nation.

DISCLOSURE

The authors have nothing to disclose.

REFERENCES

1. Dossey BM. Integrative health and wellness assessment. In: Dossey BM, Luck S, Gulino-Schaub B, editors. Nurse coaching integrative approaches for health and wellbeing. Miami (FL): International Nurse Coach Association; 2015. p. 109–21.

2. Bodenheimer T, Sinsky C. From triple aim to quadruple aim: care of the patient requires care of the provider. Ann Fam Med 2014;12:573–6.

3. Hess D, Dossey BM, Southward ME, et al. The art & science of nurse coaching. Silver Spring (MA): ANA; 2013.

4. NCCAM has a new name. NCCIH Web site. 2015. Available at: https://nccih.nih.gov/about/offices/od/nccam-new-name. Accessed October 20, 2019.

5. Complementary, alternative or integrative health, what's in a name? NICCH web site. 2018. Available at: https://nccih.nih.gov/health/integrative-health#hed1. Accessed October 20, 2019.

6. Jonas W. How healing works. New York: Lorena Jones Books; 2018.

7. Kreitzer MJ, Koithan M. Integrative nursing. New York: Oxford; 2014.

8. Guntupalli KK, Wachtel S, Mallampalli A, et al. Burnout in the intensive care unit professionals. Indian J Crit Care Med 2014;8(3):139–43.

9. Burnout the national summit on prevention and management of burnout in the ICU. Critical Care Societies Collaborative (CCSC) Web site. 2017. Available at: http://ccsconline.org/optimizing-the-workforce/burnout. Accessed October 20, 2019.

10. Panagioti M, Panagopoulou E, Bower P, et al. Controlled interventions to reduce burnout in physicians: a systematic review and meta-analysis. JAMA Int Med 2017;177(2):195–205.

11. West CP, Dyrbye LN, Erwin PJ, et al. Interventions to prevent and reduce physician burnout: a systematic review and meta-analysis. Lancet 2016;388(10057):2272–81.

12. McElligott D, Capitulo KL, Morris DL, et al. The effect of a holistic program on health promoting behaviors in hospital registered nurses. J Holist Nurs 2010; 28:175–83.
13. Healthy Nurse Healthy Nation. American Nurses Association (ANA). Web site. 2017. Available at: https://www.healthynursehealthynation.org/. Accessed October 20, 2019.
14. Whitehead D. Health promotion in nursing. A Derridean discourse analysis. Health Promot Int 2010;26:117–27.
15. American Holistic Nurses Association (AHNA). Holistic nursing: scope and standards of practice American Nurses Association. 3rd edition. Silver Springs (MD); 2019.
16. Nightingale F. Notes on nursing. What it is what it is not. (facsimile ed.). Philadelphia: J B Lippincott; 1859/1946. p. 75.
17. Watson J. Caring science as sacred science. Philadelphia: FA Davis; 2005.
18. Dossey BM. Nursing: integral, integrative, and holistic-local to global. In: Dossey BM, Keegan L, editors. Holistic nursing: a handbook for practice. 6th edition. Burlington (VT): Jones & Bartlett Learning; 2013. p. 1–57.
19. Dossey BM. Theory of integrative nurse coaching. In: Dossey BM, Luck S, Gulino-Schaub B, editors. Nurse coaching integrative approaches for health and wellbeing. Miami (FL): International Nurse Coach Association; 2015. p. 29–48.
20. McElligott D. Healing: the journey from concept to nursing practice. J Holist Nurs 2010;28:251–9.
21. McElligott D. Self development. In: Dossey BM, Luck S, Gulino-Schaub B, editors. Nurse coaching: integrative approaches for health and wellbeing. Miami (FL): International Nurse Coach Association; 2015. p. 407–17.
22. Levin JD, Reich JL. Self –reflection. In: Dossey BM, Keegan L, editors. Holistic nursing: a handbook for practice. 6th edition. Silver Springs (MD): Jones & Bartlett Learning; 2013. p. 247–59.
23. McElligott D, Eckert S, Dossey BM, et al. Instrument development of the integrative health and wellness assessment. J Holist Nurs 2017;36:374–84.
24. Prochaska JO, DiClemente CC. The stages of change. In social work tech. 2012. Available at: http://socialworktech.com/2012/01/09/stages-of-change-prochaska-diclemente/. Accessed October 4, 2019.
25. American Holistic Nurses Association stress management toolkit. AHNA Web site. Available at. https://www.ahna.org/Home/Resources/Stress-Management. Accessed October 25, 2019.

Extinguish Burnout in Critical Care Nursing

Terri L. Bogue, MSN, RN, PCNS-BC*, Robert L. Bogue, BS

KEYWORDS

- Burnout • Nurse • Health care • Critical care nursing • Employee • Resilience

KEY POINTS

- Burnout has become epidemic in health care; up to 86% of critical care nurses report at least 1 symptom of burnout.
- The symptoms of burnout include emotional exhaustion, depersonalization or cynicism, and lack of efficacy.
- Results, support, and self-care increase personal agency, while demands decrease it. Personal agency is the individual's ability to get something completed.
- Individuals, health care teams, and leadership can positively or negatively impact burnout in critical care.
- The alignment of expectations and perceived results can decrease the risk of burnout.

INTRODUCTION

The Institute for Healthcare Improvement states that, "if burnout in healthcare were described in clinical or public health terms, it might well be called an epidemic."[1] Working in a critical care unit can be particularly stressful owing to high patient morbidity and mortality, challenging daily work routines, and frequent encounters with traumatic and ethical issues.[2] When assessed using the Maslach Burnout Inventory, 43.9% of physicians reported at least 1 symptom of burnout.[3] Using the Maslach Burnout Inventory, up to 86% of critical care nurses report at least 1 symptom of burnout, with 25% to 33% of critical care nurses manifesting symptoms of severe burnout syndrome.[4]

Burnout affects all aspects of health care. Burnout impacts the mental and physical well-being of the physicians, nurses, and other health care providers and has a negative impact on their families.[4] It leads to decreased staff engagement, which correlates with a less positive patient experience, decreased productivity, and an increased risk of workplace accidents. These all significantly affect the financial vitality of the

Thor Projects LLC, 106 Jordan Court, Carmel, IN 46032, USA
* Corresponding author.
E-mail address: tbogue@thorprojects.com
Twitter: @BogueTerri (T.L.B.); @RobBogue (R.L.B.)

Crit Care Nurs Clin N Am 32 (2020) 451–463
https://doi.org/10.1016/j.cnc.2020.05.007
0899-5885/20/© 2020 Elsevier Inc. All rights reserved.
ccnursing.theclinics.com

organization. The impact on patient care is even more concerning. Lower levels of staff engagement are linked with lower quality patient care, including safety. Burnout also limits providers' empathy, a crucial component of effective and person-centered care.[1]

WHAT IS BURNOUT?

In 1974, Herbert Freudenberger first wrote about staff burnout.[5] The article explored the physical signs and behavioral indicators. In *Burn-out: The High Cost of High Achievement*, Freudenberger described individuals with burnout as "their inner resources are consumed as if by fire, leaving a great emptiness inside, although their outer shells may be more or less unchanged." Freudenberger further commented, "Burn-out is pretty much limited to dynamic, charismatic, goal-oriented men and women or to determined idealists who want their marriages to be the best, their work records to be outstanding, their children to shine, their community to be better." From the beginning of the literature, Freudenberger associated burnout with aspirations for accomplishments.[6]

Freudenberger defined burnout as "a wearing out, exhaustion, or failure resulting from excessive demands made on energy, strength, or resources."[7] The core of these original descriptions continues today; burnout is most commonly described by exhaustion, cynicism, and inefficacy. Examining the details of the components of burnout provides additional insight.

Emotional exhaustion increases as emotional resources are depleted and workers feel they are no longer able to give of themselves at a psychological level. For example, a worker may encounter this feeling of exhaustion, specifically emotional exhaustion, when providing care to a patient who has little hope of survival.

Depersonalization is a distant or indifferent attitude toward work. This is sometimes referred to as "disengagement." It manifests as negative, callous, and cynical behaviors or interactions with colleagues or patients in an impersonal manner. Depersonalization may be expressed as unprofessional comments directed toward coworkers, blaming patients for their medical problems, or the inability to express empathy or grief when a patient dies.

Decreased feelings of effectiveness and a lack of accomplishments are derived from the tendency to negatively evaluate the value of one's work, feelings of insufficiency regarding the ability to perform one's job, and a poor professional self-esteem.[8]

UNDERSTANDING BURNOUT

It may be possible to identify burnout based on its definition; however, this is not particularly helpful in preventing or recovering from it. The key to being able to prevent or recover from burnout is found through understanding the factors that enhance and those that deplete personal agency. The Bathtub Model and the Expectations–Results Gap Model enable the individual to more easily identify areas where they may have opportunities to become more resilient to burnout.

Bathtub Model

A visual and more easily assimilated view of burnout can be found in the Bathtub Model **(Fig. 1)**.[9] The perception of personal agency provides each person the actual ability to get something completed. It is the sum of the time available to do things and the individual's physical and emotional ability to get them done. Personal agency is represented by water in the bathtub in the Bathtub Model. Personal agency is filled by some activities and thought processes, and it is depleted by demands. By regulating these inputs and outputs, it is possible to maintain or regain personal agency. Each of the inputs and the

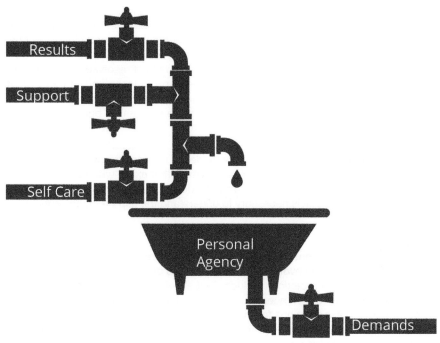

Fig. 1. Bathtub Model

output can be regulated, like a valve on a pipe regulates the flow through that pipe. It is necessary to examine the components that increase personal agency and those that decrease it to obtain a better understanding of the process of burnout.

The first source that increases personal agency is results. Results create resources in terms of material resources, social capital, and skills that make it possible to accomplish more. Results allow individuals, over time, to strive for greater goals, having overcome previous hurdles and having developed the internal and external rewards for those results.[9]

The second source that increases personal agency is support. Support is the resource that others provide and can be leveraged to affect change. Support is most impactful when the nurse is aware of it, accepts it, and recognizes how their success is supported by others.[9] There are 3 kinds of support available to individuals: emotional support, material support, and systemic support. Emotional support is found when the individual feels loved or cared for. Material support may be financial, shared work or responsibility, or other physical items provided to make the individual's world a bit easier. Finally, systemic support is found in structures that make processes and work easier and more productive.[9]

The third source that increases personal agency is self-care; of the 3 sources that increase personal agency, self-care is the only one that both increases personal agency and expands the capacity for personal agency in the individual. Self-care includes not only physical self-care activities such as exercise, nutrition, hydration, and rest, but also psychological self-care activities, including positive self-talk, an integrated self-image, and rejuvenating actions.[9]

The drain of the bathtub illustrates the impact of demands that the individual has or perceives they have. Although often understood as externally generated, many demands are internally generated based on external demands. Establishing decision-making criteria for accepting new demands and boundaries for external demands that will be rejected are important components of managing the demands that individuals allow. In addition, evaluating demands to see if the effort is greater than the received rewards can expose a "trade imbalance" that may be best resolved by rejecting the demand. Further, a change in mindset from pessimistic to optimistic can mitigate the impact of demands. As the individual becomes more adept at managing demands to reserve their personal agency, they become more resistant to burnout.[9]

The Expectations–Results Gap

Although the Bathtub Model is an effective model for making burnout understandable, it is limited in its ability to illustrate the discontinuity that exists when burnout occurs. Frequently, those exhibiting burnout symptoms describe a defining event as a "snap." To understand this snap, it is necessary to understand the gap between expectations and perceived results.

Expectations

One of the primary functions of the human brain is its predictive capacity. It has been theorized that humor is an evolutionary adaptation to detect and correct errors in this predictive capacity.[10] Predictions include the behavior of others, environmental factors, and the predictor's own agency. An individual's predictions of their own agency are converted into expectations for themselves and their capacity to accomplish objectives. However, predictions are subject to numerous biases, heuristics, and effects, including imaginability bias, confirmation bias, priming effect, the halo effect, and the framing effect.[11] These biases may cause the expectations of the individual to be unrealistic.

Perceived results

The perception of an individual's results may be influenced by the feedback they receive about those results. This feedback can be accurate, inaccurate, or nonexistent. Inaccurate or nonexistent feedback can lead to a misperception of the actual results. This may result in a greater—or, more frequently, diminished—sense of results.

Where possible, individuals should seek to calibrate their perception of results with reality through active solicitation of feedback and the use of trusted feedback channels.

The gap

Burnout is felt when an event occurs, during which the individual assesses the gap between their expectations and perceived results and finds the gap to be too large. The event need not be a major life event, yet they may find during their assessment that they did not meet their expectations for efficacy.

The sudden realization of this gap may result in feelings of inefficacy and therefore a lack of control. This lack of control was first expressed by Martin Seligman and Steve Meier as "learned helplessness."[12] Subsequent neurologic research made it clear that it was not helplessness that was learned but instead control, and this learned control dampens the default, helplessness response.[13]

BURNOUT IN CRITICAL CARE

Working in critical care can be especially stressful because of the high patient morbidity and mortality, challenging daily work routines, and regular encounters with traumatic and ethical issues.[4] The level of nearly continuous care provided to the patients and the stress from constantly changing conditions can result in the perception that there is not enough time or resources to provide proper care to the patients. The impact of the critical care environment is that health care providers practicing in critical care have one of the highest rates of burnout at 50%.[4]

The critical care environment may have some of the highest prevalence of burnout, but not all critical care units have a high incidence of burnout. The environment of the unit and hospital has a direct impact on the prevalence of burnout. Units where the critical care nurses report the highest prevalence of burnout among their colleagues were more likely to have burnout themselves.[4] The opposite of this is true as well. The units where the critical care nurse reports few incidents of burnout in their colleagues are also less likely to report burnout themselves. Studies show that the most common work-related factors related to burnout are exclusion from the decision-making process, the need for greater autonomy, security risks, and staffing issues.[14] When units develop standards that address these factors in a positive way, the impact and work-related stress is reduced.

RISK FACTORS COMMON TO CRITICAL CARE NURSES

The Bathtub Model demonstrates that a lack of personal agency is a ticket to the world of burnout.[9] Synthesizing the literature and reviewing the risk factors for burnout related to the critical care nurse results in the outline of four categories of risk factors for burnout: personal characteristics, organizational factors, quality of working relationships, and exposure to end-of-life issues. Each of these categories are broken down into subcategories that increase the risk for burnout (**Fig. 2**).[4]

Identifying specifics for each of the categories of risk factors for burnout allows the nurse to understand the impact on their personal agency. This understanding is necessary in the prevention and recovery from burnout.

Personal Characteristics

The first personal characteristic that increases the risk of burnout is self-criticism. The way individuals talk to themselves about themselves is frequently filled with criticism and shame.[15] Too frequently, individuals speak to themselves in a way they would never speak to another human being. When individuals condemn their own actions and berate themselves for the smallest infraction, they begin to believe that they are not good enough or they are not providing the care they should to the patient.[9] Self-criticism changes the perceived results of the care they provide. Others may provide feedback that the care the individual provided was incredible; however, individuals with high degrees of self-criticism may be unable to accept this feedback.

In addition to self-criticism, the utilization of unhealthy coping strategies increases the likelihood of burnout. Coping strategies are activities that help the individual deal with constantly changing cognitive and behavioral efforts necessary to manage specific external and/or internal demands that are considered taxing or exceeding the resources of the individual.[16] The utilization of unhealthy coping strategies, including denial, depersonalization, compartmentalization, suppression, social isolation, and substance abuse, can result in negative long-term consequences.[17]

The lack of both physical and psychological self-care further increases the risk of burnout. Physical self-care, including diet, exercise, hydration, and sleep, is critical to the prevention of burnout. The individual may consider the time it takes to perform self-care an indulgence that they should be doing for others. However, the evidence is clear that self-care is imperative to one's emotional health.[18]

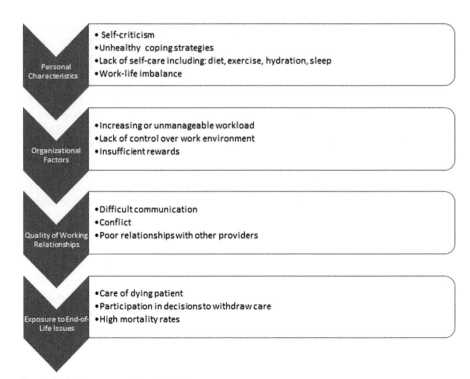

Personal Characteristics
- Self-criticism
- Unhealthy coping strategies
- Lack of self-care including: diet, exercise, hydration, sleep
- Work-life imbalance

Organizational Factors
- Increasing or unmanageable workload
- Lack of control over work environment
- Insufficient rewards

Quality of Working Relationships
- Difficult communication
- Conflict
- Poor relationships with other providers

Exposure to End-of-Life Issues
- Care of dying patient
- Participation in decisions to withdraw care
- High mortality rates

Fig. 2. Risk factors associated with burnout.

The final personal characteristic that is a risk factor for burnout is the presence of a work-life imbalance. It can be difficult to identify a work-life imbalance in oneself, particularly if there is currently an imbalance. Understanding the key indicators of a work-life imbalance facilitates recognizing such an imbalance. Some of the key indicators include skipping meals, eating a poorly balanced diet, working through an entire shift without any breaks, arriving home late from work, difficulty sleeping, sleeping less than 5 hours per night, changing personal or family plans because of work, and feeling frustrated by technology (**Fig. 3**).[19] Ensuring work-life balance is an important step to reducing the risk of burnout.

Organizational Factors

Like individuals, organizations have specific factors that can increase the risk of burnout for their employees. An increasing or unmanageable workload is an organizational risk factor for burnout. An overloaded work schedule, described as having too little time to complete one's work and too few resources to accomplish the job, is a major source of burnout.[20] The increasing workload in critical care is exacerbated by high patient morbidity and mortality, challenging daily work routines, and regular encounters with traumatic and moral or ethical issues. The results of this increased workload can rapidly accelerate when providers perceive that there is insufficient time or limited resources to properly care for their patients.[4]

A lack of control over the work environment is an organizational risk factor for burnout. The nurse's involvement in hospital and unit policies and their ability to influence decisions is not only important for professional satisfaction, it is also an antidote for burnout and stimulates engagement.[21]

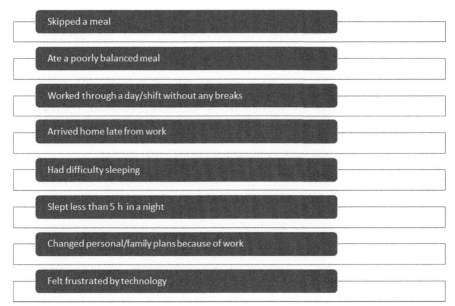

Fig. 3. Indicators of work–life imbalance.

Insufficient rewards are the final organizational risk factor for burnout. Meaningful recognition is a significant predictor of decreased burnout and higher employee satisfaction.[22] A key tenet of the American Association of Critical Care Nurses' Healthy Work Environment Standards is "a recognition system that reaches from the bedside to the boardroom, ensuring individuals receive recognition consistent with their personal definition of meaning, fulfillment, development, and advancement at every stage of their professional career".[23]

Quality of Working Relationships

Relationships among coworkers can provide a great deal of social support when employees have effective means of working out disagreements.

The quality of working relationships impacts the expectations and cultural norms of the unit, which, in turn, impact the work-life climate and expectations for individual work-life balance. The work-life climate of the unit impacts the work-life balance of the individual nurses on the unit and is one of the strongest associations with burnout climate and personal burnout.[19]

Individuals who are experiencing burnout can have a negative impact on their colleagues by causing greater personal conflict and disrupting job tasks. In this way, burnout can become contagious and perpetuate itself through social interactions on the job.[24]

Exposure to End-of-Life Issues

Risk factors related to end-of-life issues include caring for a dying patient and participating in or witnessing decisions to forego life-sustaining treatments. It is important to acknowledge that units with higher mortality rates have been associated with increased rates of burnout.[4]

IMPACT OF BURNOUT ON THE CRITICAL CARE NURSE

Overall, 40% of hospital nurses have burnout levels that exceed the norms for health care workers.[25] Burnout in critical care providers may result in post-traumatic stress disorder (PTSD), alcohol or substance abuse, and even suicidal ideation.[4] PTSD is manifested with intrusion, avoidance, negative alterations in cognition and mood, and marked alteration in arousal and reactivity. PTSD can occur in response to one catastrophic event or after chronic or repetitive exposure to traumatic episodes. Between 22% to 29% of critical care nurses have symptoms of PTSD, and up to 18% of critical care nurses meet the diagnostic criteria for PTSD. Additionally, 98% of nurses with PTSD will also have symptoms consistent with burnout.[2]

Impact on Critical Care Patients

Burnout affects health care providers with a frequency that is concerning. Nurse burnout impacts far more people than the nurses themselves. Burnout among nurses may contribute to a reduced quality of care, increased number of medical errors, higher rates of health care-associated infections, decreased patient safety, and higher 30-day mortality rates.[4] The emotional exhaustion among burned out nurses can increase the likelihood that patients will rate a hospital poorly, refuse to recommend hospitals for care, and perceive nurse communications unfavorably.[26] These patient satisfaction indicators can have a negative impact on the hospital's reputation and reimbursement as well as the nurse's perception of the care they provide.

Impact on Health Care

There are many factors that influence a health care professional's decision to leave their current position, one of which is burnout. Job dissatisfaction among hospital nurses is four times greater than the average for all workers in the United States, and one in four hospital nurses report that they intend to leave their current jobs within 1 year.[25] Employee turnover is expensive. The cost of replacing one critical care nurse is estimated to be more than $65,000.[4] There is more involved in increasing nurse turnover than the cost of replacing nurses; excessive turnover increases health care costs, decreases productivity, lowers staff morale, and reduces the overall quality of care. The reduction in quality of care is closely related to the loss of experienced professionals leaving critical care, who must then be replaced, frequently with less experience professionals. Turnover among critical care nurses ranges between 13% to 20% per year, while the US average turnover for all types of employees is only 10.4%. In one survey, 22% of nurses planned to leave their professions. When asked why they were considering leaving nursing, 56% stated they wanted a less stressful position.[4]

TOOLS AND TECHNIQUES FOR RECOVERING FROM AND PREVENTING BURNOUT

While diagnostic criteria and impact assessments are essential for understanding the scope of the problem, the key opportunity is found in helping staff recover from burnout and building a culture that is burnout resistant.

Individuals

Individuals who suffer from burnout or wish to prevent burnout have two key tools. First, they can focus on appropriate self-care. Second, they can anchor expectations and their perception of their results in reality. Ultimately, it is the individual who is suffering, and it is therefore the individual who must invest in taking the steps necessary to recover.

Self-care
Nurses tend to believe that self-care is unnecessary or self-indulgent. They fail to recognize the wisdom of the Federal Aviation Administration mandated safety announcements, which state "put your own mask on before helping others." The key issue with self-care is helping nurses accept that it is a necessity and not a nicety. Changing the perception from self-care as stealing time or care from others to an attitude of additional efficacy that a nurse has is directly related to their ability and willingness to do self-care.

Physical self-care is necessary to provide the care the nurse desires to provide to their patient. Physical exercise is related to significant improvements in mood and reductions in confusion, anger, and tension.[27] Small, simple, and sustainable changes can increase physical activity and lead to a reduced chance of entering burnout.[28] Proper nutrition is a major factor in influencing personal health and reducing the effects of stress and inflammation on the body.[29] Often, adults fall short of the recommended daily intake for water of 2700 to 3700 mL. This range reflects differences in gender and activity level. While severe dehydration can be a life-threatening event, the effects of mild dehydration are frequently overlooked. These symptoms of mild dehydration can include fatigue, confusion, and anger.[30] Of all the physical self-care activities available, the strongest linkage to teamwork and safety involve adequate sleep.[19]

Psychological self-care is as important as physical self-care. Utilizing positive self-talk rather than negative self-talk interrupts a pattern of unconscious negative and self-critical thoughts. This allows the individual to tap into a sense of confidence about handling a situation, and it can also relax the body and improve overall mood.[31]

Grounding
Grounding both expectations and results in reality minimizes the potential for gaps and therefore for triggering burnout. Expectations should be assessed in relation to prior experiences as well as norms for other people in similar roles and situations. Individuals frequently fail to recognize the degree to which the environment they are in influences their capacity to get things done.

The most common challenge with calibrating the perception of results is the failure to receive any feedback. Where possible, designing feedback mechanisms to ensure that nurses can see the outcomes for the patients they care for should be encouraged. Even in units with high mortality, the reality of the outcome will frequently be less destressing than not knowing.[17]

Teams and Peers
Health care is a "team sport."[32] Teams can either discourage or encourage burnout. The cultural norms of the team when shaped around support and demands management can be effective barriers to burnout.

Support
While leadership has a role in providing support for nurses, the greatest support comes from the relationship with the other members of the health care team in the unit.[33] Team members who are concerned for their peers can intentionally shape the culture by actively offering support when they can and responding to the requests for assistance from their peers. Recognizing emotional exhaustion and burnout in peers and stepping in to provide support builds a culture in which a burnout climate cannot thrive and staff thrives.[19]

Demands

Patient acuity is always a variable in nursing care. Patients who are relatively stable one moment can require emergent care in a moment. Even if nursing assignments are equitable over the period of a shift, they will not be equal at any given moment. Teams that work individually to get their patients caught up so that they have a capacity to help their peers in times of peak demand do not experience demands as intensely as units in which helping is not as common.

Leadership

Leadership plays a multi-dimensional role in discouraging burnout on their units. Their role in advocating for the units and shaping the culture of team members toward helping one another contributes to better outcomes for the nurses they lead.

Support

Recognizing the challenges and impact of high workload in distressing patient situations is necessary to develop ways to adjust time with complicated and difficult patients and families, support for work-life balance, and the acceptance of mental health days to refresh the staff's reserves.[17] Providing additional resources and support during times of high unit mortality can help reduce the impact of caring for dying patients and their families. It is necessary to develop a sustainable and manageable workload for staff that provides opportunities to use and refine existing skills as well as become effective in new skills to provide a culture that minimizes burnout.[2]

In addition to supporting staff in dealing with distressing situations, it is necessary to not only include staff in unit decisions but also to support their participation on unit and facility shared governance committees. This participation provides the opportunity to have influence on their work and the work environment, increasing engagement.[24]

Results

While difficult patient care situations occur every day in the critical care environment, it is important for staff to know the positive result of the care they provide.[17] Feedback to staff about patients who have survived and even thrived is crucial to create a realistic view of the staff's results and dispel the perception that their work is not important, and few patients survive and return to normal.

Providing consistency in rewards between the person and the work they do means that there are both material rewards and opportunities for intrinsic satisfaction.[24] This helps increase the feelings of results for a job well done and greater self-efficacy.

Self-care

Subtle cues often send powerful messages to nurses. Leaders who neglect their own self-care send a message that self-care is not important. A tangible area of concern is the degree to which nurses take their lunch breaks.[34] Lunch breaks are essential self-care for everyone. In critical care nursing, it is not always possible to take a lunch break. However, it should be normal to take lunch breaks, and only in extreme cases should these be skipped. Leaders can model the behavior and even support the unit when necessary to ensure that nurses are able to take a lunch break, even if it must be abbreviated.

Demands

The development of thoughtful staffing approaches that provide an appropriately trained nurse for each patient and consider the emotional impact to the nurse of managing challenging or distressing patients over multiple shifts helps to manage the demands of high workloads that drive burnout.[17] Supporting an appropriate work-life balance promotes staff who are more engaged in the work setting, adaptable to changing team dynamics, appropriately resolve conflicts, and proactively promote safety at work.[19]

SUMMARY

Burnout has become widespread among health care providers; approximately 40% of nurses in hospitals experience burnout at levels that exceed the norm for health care providers.[25] The impact of burnout extends far beyond the individuals suffering from burnout; the entire health care team and their patients are negatively affected.

Burnout is identified as a combination of exhaustion, cynicism, and a lack of efficacy. The Bathtub Model is a visual model that describes the sources that increase personal agency as results, support, and self-care. Each of these help the individual to be more resistant to burnout. The Bathtub Model also includes the impact of demands in draining the individual's personal agency. Controlling the flow of results, support, self-care and demands provides the control to reduce the risk of burnout.

The Expectations-Results Gap Model can provide a different view of where burnout originates. When the individual's expectations are not aligned with their perceived results, the gap found is where burnout originates from. Finding methods to maintain realistic expectations and recognition of results further reduces or eliminates burnout.[9]

Individual characteristics can increase the risk for burnout. These factors include negative self-talk, the use of unhealthy coping strategies, a lack of physical and psychological self-care, and the presence of a work-life imbalance. There are also organizational characteristics that are responsible for some of the factors that cause burnout. These factors, frequently experienced in critical care, include an overloaded work schedule, a lack of control over the work environment, and insufficient rewards. Stressful or high conflict relationships with coworkers also increases the risk for burnout. Finally, exposure to end of life issues, which can be common in critical care, is a risk factor for burnout.[4]

Recognizing the causes and risk factors of burnout is helpful, but it is more important to be able to utilize the tools and techniques that make recovery from or prevention of burnout possible. Individuals need to commit to both physical and psychological self-care, be willing to receive support, and recognize their results. These tools, combined with managing demands, can create the opportunity to escape burnout.

Health care teams can develop a unit where support is offered and accepted as the norm while balancing the demands in a way that the patients are well cared for and the staff share the burden.

Leaders need to provide the necessary support for staff to deliver quality to their patients. This is possible through thoughtful and innovating staffing and balancing workloads. Leaders are in a unique position that allows them to identify the positive results of individuals and the team and provide rewards in a meaningful way. Finally, leaders need to be examples to their staff of the importance of physical and psychological self-care. This sets the tone for everyone on the unit.

Experiencing the hollow pain of burnout occurs too frequently among health care providers. Taking the time for self-care, accepting support, recognizing the positive results of one's actions combined with managing demands can protect individuals from experiencing burnout.

DISCLOSURE

The authors also wrote the book *Extinguish Burnout: A Practical Guide to Prevention and Recovery*. They do not believe this to be a conflict of interest.

REFERENCES

1. Perlo J, Balik B, Swensen S, et al. IHI framework for improving joy in work. Cambridge (MA): Institute for Healthcare Improvement; 2017.
2. Mealer M, Moss M, Good V, et al. What is burnout syndrome (BOS). Am J Respir Crit Care Med 2016;194:1–2.
3. Shanafelt T, West C, Sinsky C, et al. Changes in Burnout and Satisfaction With Work-Life Integration in Physicians and the General US Working Population Between 2011 and 2017. Mayo Clinic Proceedings 2019;94(9):1681–94.
4. Moss M, Good V, Gozal D, et al. An official critical care societies collaborative statement: burnout syndrome in critical care healthcare professionals: a call for action. Crit Care Med 2016;44(7):14–21.
5. Freudenberger HJ. Staff burn-out. J Soc Issues 1974;30(1).
6. Freudenberger HJ. Burn-out: the high cost of high achievement. New York: Bantam Books, Inc; 1980.
7. Freudenberger HJ. Burn-out: occupational hazard of the child care worker. Child Care Q 1977;6:90.
8. Maslach C, Jackson E, Leiter P. Maslach burnout inventory. 3rd edition. Palo Alto (CA): Consulting Psychologists Press; 1997.
9. Bogue R, Bogue T. Extinguish burnout a practical guide to prevention and recovery. Alexandria (VA): Society of Human Resource Management; 2019.
10. Hurley MM, Dennett DC, Adams RB Jr. Inside jokes: using humor to reverse-engineer the mind. Cambridge (MA): The MIT Press; 2011.
11. Kahneman D. Thinking, fast and slow. New York: Farrar, Strauss, and Giroux; 2011.
12. Seligman MEP, Maier SF. Failure to escape traumatic shock. J Exp Psychol 1967; 74:1–9.
13. Maier SF, Seligman MEP. Learned helplessness at fifty: insights from neuroscience. Psychol Rev 2016;123(4):349–67.
14. The Joint Commission. Developing resilience to combat nurse burnout. Oakbrook Terrace (IL): The Joint Commission; 2019. Quick Safety.
15. Brown B. Daring Greatly: How the Courage to Be Vulnerable Transforms the Way We Live, Love, Parent, and Lead. New York: Penguin Random House; 2012.
16. Shin H, Park YM, Ying JY, et al. Relationships between coping strategies and burnout symptoms: a meta-analytic approach. Prof Psychol Res Pr 2014;4(1): 44–56.
17. Costa DK, Moss M. The cost of caring: emotion, burnout, and psychological distress in critical care clinicians. Ann Am Thorac Soc 2018;15(7):787–90.
18. Richards K. The power of self-care to transform culture, improve retention, and boost resilience. Nurse Leader 2014;12(1):57–9.
19. Schwartz SP, Adair KC, Bae J, et al. Work-life balance behaviours cluster in work settings and relate to burnout and safety culture: a cross-sectional survey analysis. BMJ Qual Saf 2018;28:142–50.
20. Laschinger HKS, Leiter M. The impact of nursing work environments on patient safety outcomes: the mediating role of burnout. J Nurs Adm 2006;36:259–67.
21. Van Bogaert P, Meulemans H, Clarke S, et al. Hospital nurse practice environment, burnout, job outcomes and quality of care: test of a structural equation model. J Adv Nurs 2009;65(10):2175–85.
22. Kelly LA, Lefton C. Effect of meaningful recognition on critical care nurses' compassion fatigue. Am J Crit Care 2017;26:438–44.

23. American Association of Critical Care Nurses. Meaningful recognition. Aliso Viejo, CA: American Association of Critical Care Nurses; 2019. Available at: https://www.aacn.org/nursing-excellence/healthy-work-environments/meaningful-recognition. Accessed October 15, 2019.

24. Maslach C, Leiter M. Understanding the burnout experience: recent research and its implications for psychiatry. World Psychiatry 2016;15(2):103–11.

25. Aiken LH, Clarke SP, Sloane DM, et al. Hospital nurse staffing and patient mortality, nurse burnout, and job dissatisfaction. J Am Med Assoc 2002;288(16):1987–93.

26. Dyrbye LN, West CP, Johnson PO, et al. Burnout and satisfaction with work-life integration among nurses. J Occup Environ Med 2019;61(8):689–98.

27. Penedo FJ, Dahn JR. Exercise and well-being: a review of mental and physical benefits associated with physical activity. Curr Opin Psychiatry 2005;18(2):189–93.

28. Deutschman A. Change or die. New York: Harper Collins; 2009.

29. Criscitelli T. Influencing optimum health for nurses. AORN J 2017;105(2):228–31.

30. Popkin BM, D'Anci KE, Rosenberg IH. Water, hydration, and health. Nutr Rev 2010;68(8):439–58.

31. Crane PJ, Ward SF. Self-healing and self-care for nurses. AORN J 2016;104:386–400.

32. Pearl R. Mistreated: why we think we're getting good health care-and why we're usually wrong. New York,: PublicAffairs; 2017.

33. Apker J, Propp K, Zabava Ford WS. Investigating the effect of nurse-team communication on nurse turnover: relationships among communication processes, identification, and intent to leave. Health Commun 2009;24:106–14.

34. Witkoski A, Vaughan Dickson V. Hospital staff nurses' work hours, meal periods, and rest breaks. A review from an occupational health nurse perspective. AAOHN J 2010;58(11):489–97.

Self-Achievement Through Creativity in Critical Care

Susan Bartos, PhD, RN, CCRN

KEYWORDS

- Self-actualization • Creativity • Empathy • Critical care

KEY POINTS

- Creativity and various mediums of artistic expressions can be used as a restorative self-care practice.
- Regular practices in creativity aid in boosting empathy and empathic behaviors in health care providers.
- Critical care units are a lush environment for innovation and creativity and nurses should seek creative opportunities to achieve self-actualization.

Art in nursing is present in various forms and there is ample literature exploring topics of creativity including journaling for clinicians,[1] intensive care unit (ICU) diaries for patients and providers,[2,3] and music therapy for patients.[4] Illness narratives, depictions of the sick, or the effects of disease are commonly represented in media or through various expressions of creativity. This article highlights how creativity and various mediums of artistic expressions may can be used as a self-care practice and may aid in boosting empathy and empathic behaviors in health care providers. Theories on empathy are presented, as well as selected representations of nursing as creative expressions and the importance of promoting creativity and empathy especially in the critical care environment.

BACKGROUND

Self-care was defined by the World Health Organization first in 2009 and the definition continues to be updated as, "the ability of individuals, families and communities to promote health, prevent disease, maintain health, and cope with illness and disability with or without the support of a health-care provider."[5] Recently, self-care and self-care practices have gained in popularity as an intervention for chronic health care conditions and syndromes such as heart failure,[6] diabetes mellitus,[7] chronic obstructive pulmonary disease,[8] and chronic kidney disease.[9] There is ample literature to support

Egan School of Nursing, Fairfield University, 1073 North Benson Road, Fairfield, CT 06824, USA
E-mail address: sbartos@fairfield.edu
Twitter: @Prof_SBar (S.B.)

Crit Care Nurs Clin N Am 32 (2020) 465–472
https://doi.org/10.1016/j.cnc.2020.05.004
0899-5885/20/© 2020 Elsevier Inc. All rights reserved.

self-care practices for caregivers[10] and as a way for well individuals to adopt as a way of daily living.

Although self-care and its practices are at the cornerstone of many disease management programs, many self-care interventions are also designed to keep one in a state of well-being. These self-care practices—eating a balanced diet, sleeping the recommended number of hours per night, exercising, and maintaining a sound and sensible mind—are often simple and extrinsic-based measures one may take to live well, but do not elevate self-care to a level of meaning and purpose.[11]

Aristotle wrote of the highest aim for humanity, a concept he called "eudaimonia," as both living well and doing well. One may find eudaimonia in different ways, but it is important to separate quick, simple pleasures (hedonic) from virtuosic and gratifying habits. The quest for happiness, true happiness and not happiness for the sake of being happy, is another consideration. Living a balanced life, a wise life, a virtuous life, are the ways to self-fulfillment.[12]

Within health care, and particularly critical care, clinician and nurse well-being remains a pressing concern. Emotional exhaustion, depersonalization, and reduced personal accomplishment, a cluster of symptoms better known as "burnout," affect up to 86% of critical care nurses and occurs when the individual's expectations from oneself differ from those of the organization's expectations.[13] In a statement[14] from the Critical Care Collaboratives Society (American Association of Critical Care Nurses, American College of Chest Physicians, the American Thoracic Society, and the Society of Critical Care Medicine) risk factors to identify individuals at greatest risk for burnout syndrome were identified. These characteristics include those who have a high level of idealism, perfectionism, and who are overcommitted, with difficulties in establishing a work–life balance and boundaries.[14] Performing recommended, holistic, self-care behaviors that tend to the body, the mind, and the spirit may help to mitigate the effects of burnout syndrome.[14] These measures, although important and foundational, should be augmented with interventions that instill a sense of fulfillment in the practitioner.

Fulfilment and self-achievement sit atop the hierarchy of human needs. Abraham Maslow first defined this concept (1954) and continued to refine the theory (1968) throughout his studies of human psychology. Maslow presents human needs as a pyramid (**Fig. 1**) with the highest priority needs as the foundation of the structure. Should these needs not be met, the individual will have difficulty moving up and through the hierarchy. Self-achievement is located at the top of the pyramid, only accessible when the rest of the basic human needs have been satisfied. One way to self-actualization is through a creative or moral life. Self-achievement is accomplished when the individual becomes who they desire to be, the best version of themselves.[15]

EMPATHY

Empathy is the ability to understand and share the feelings of another,[16] and a foundation of nursing and health care. Yet, there are health care providers who choose to care for others without ever having needed to be cared for. Perhaps this person may have known someone who was under the care of another or was motivated to enter a career in health care for another reason, but the development of empathy is integral to a caring and wise practitioner. Art and creative works are ways to expand the understanding and the sharing of feelings of each other, fostering the feelings of empathy between patient and provider. In Virginia Wolfe's opening sentence of her essay, "On Being Ill," she questions why more novels and literature are not focused on the common human experience of being in an illness state,

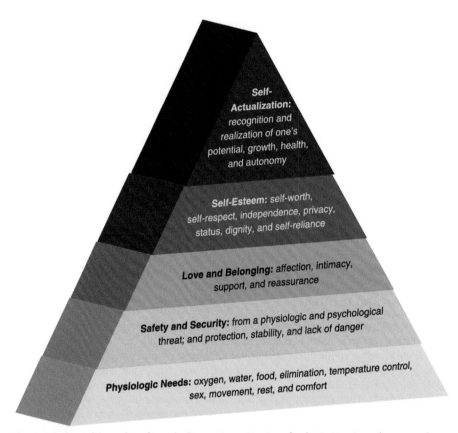

Fig. 1. Maslow's hierarchy of needs. (*From* Yoost BL, Crawford, LR. Nursing, theory, and professional practice. In: Fundamentals of nursing: active learning for collaborative practice, 2nd ed. St. Louis: Elsevier; 2020. p. 11; with permission.)

Considering how common illness is, how tremendous the spiritual change that it brings, how astonishing, when the lights of health go down, the undiscovered countries that are then disclosed, what wastes and deserts of the soul a slight attack of influenza brings to light, what precipices and lawns sprinkled with bright flowers a little rise of temperature reveals, what ancient and obdurate oaks are uprooted in us in the act of sickness, how we go down into the pit of death and feel the waters of annihilation close above our heads and wake thinking to find ourselves in the presence of angels and the harpers when we have a tooth out and come to the surface in the dentist's arm chair and confuse his 'Rise the mouth-rinse the mouth' with the greeting of the Deity stooping from the floor of Heaven to welcome us- when we think of this and infinitely more, as we are so frequently forced to think of it, it becomes strange indeed that illness has not taken its place with love, battle, and jealousy among the prime themes of literature.

The opening lines of this sentence eloquently capture the human bond of illness. Creativity fosters empathic behaviors, just as empathic behaviors can foster creative practices. Interpreting lived experiences through metaphorical speech, narrative accounts, or visual representations is validating for both the artist and the individual viewing the art. When the art is focused around the topic of illness, health care, or nursing, comfort may be found through the shared interpretative experience. Physical experiences, including the sensory experience, facilitate future decision making[17] and support future creative practices.

Postintensive care syndrome (PICS) is a cluster of symptoms that persist after the person has left the ICU and can involve the body and the thoughts, and can affect the friends and family of the individual who experienced the critical illness.[14] PICS has been studied a variety of settings, including the neurointensive care unit[18] and in pediatrics.[19] Symptoms of PICS can vary, but may include muscle weakness, difficulty with concentrating or thinking, uncontrollable anxiety or depression, or nightmares.[20]

PICS remains a condition characterized as resistant and difficult to identify early.[21,22] Alleviating the symptoms of PICS and increasing staff satisfaction are the purposes of an ICU diary.[2,23] Nurses and family caregivers[23] who participated in the keeping of an ICU diary for patients reported higher empathy levels[2] and higher satisfaction with their nursing role, yet there is conflicting evidence to support whether the use of an ICU diary helps to mitigate symptoms of post-traumatic stress disorder after a stay in the ICU.[22] Implementing a photo diary may have different effects[22] and may encourage a different expression of creativity in the ICU environment.

INNOVATION AND CREATIVITY

Nursing is portrayed in many forms of art and creativity including paintings, sculptures, photography, and television and film. Nurses are also the drivers of innovative change. The everyday equipment or processes within the hospital setting were born from the mind of a nurse, including the cardiac arrest crash cart (Anita Dorr, 1968), bilirubin lights for neonates (Sister Jean Ward, 1950), and ostomy bags (Elise Sorensen, 1954) (Table 1). These solutions may have been created out of necessity; however, they were produced from an empathetic person, searching for a practical solution. Building on the work of Martha Rogers and her theory of accelerating change, Martha Alligood tested this theory and investigated the relationships among creativity, actualization, and empathy.[24] In certain age groups, such as those aged 18 to 60 years, creativity and empathy are positively correlated.[24] Given the average age of the American nurse is 51 years of age,[25] nurses are practicing during peak times of both empathetic and creative moments. Encouraging developing nurses to think creatively will inspire future innovation and advancements in nursing. Because teaching creativity is in itself an innovation, nursing faculty should be also be given the appropriate strategies to develop self-efficacy in developing curiosity and teaching creativity.[26] It is

Table 1	
Inventions by registered nurses	
Invention	**Nurse**
Feeding tube for veterans	Bessie Blount Griffin
Ostomy pouch	Georgann Carrubba
Neonatal phototherapy	Sister Jean Ward
Cardiac crash cart	Anita Dorr
Disposable bottle liner	Adda May Allen
Color-coded IV tubing	Teri Barton-Salinas
Cooling vest	Jill Byrne
Omphalocele dressings	Roxana Reyna

important for the critical care nurse to use creativity and innovation for the benefit to both the profession and those for whom are being cared.

CREATIVITY (AND ITS LIMITS) IN THE INTENSIVE CARE UNIT

Evidence-based nursing protocols are common and guide practice in the ICU. Protocols for managing delirium,[27] preventing catheter-associated urinary tract infections[28] or pressure ulcers,[29] and promoting early mobilization[30] exist to standardize care and optimize patient outcomes. The nurse practicing in the ICU should find methods of combining creativity into daily practice along with using protocols and safety checklist to promote the continued development of both empathy and innovation.

A method such as problem-based learning[31] to train new nurses, or for continuing education for licensed nurses, is one way to promote creativity and meta-cognitive awareness. The value of creativity has been discussed in the context of medical student education[32] and should be expanded into the education of interprofessional colleagues. Expanding education outside of traditional methods to challenge the learner to problem solve and to think differently may enable the establishment of additional imaginative innovations.

A conflict in exercising creativity may arise in the critical care unit when protocols drive daily practice and there is little to no room for creativity. Freedom to adapt practices vary, but organizations should implement nurse-driven protocols for common ICU situations, such as mechanical ventilator weaning.[22] Within these protocols, nurses should look for opportunities to individualize and infuse creative practices into the care of the critically ill person. These may include the use of music, visualization, writing, reading, or engaging the senses in a way that is safe and supportive to the ICU environment.

CREATIVITY IN NURSING

Nurses and health care providers have authored many written works capturing the unique experience of illness (**Table 2**). Translating the illness experience into the written word communicates the shared experience of being ill, of recovery, or allows the reader to understand a health care provider portrayed as a fictional character. Poetry or prose provide a vehicle for validation, for conversation, and to capture an emotion which may have been otherwise quantified or perhaps even disregarded.

Sharing in the experience from a health care provider perspective offers an open narrative from a closed perspective. Nurses and other health care providers may find validation in the words of colleagues. Patients or family members may enter the provider's narrative and appreciate the alternative perspective. The majority of individuals are born into the health care system and have an experience with the health care

Table 2 Written works by registered nurses	
Nurse	**Genre**
Jeanne LeVasseur PhD, APRN	Poetry
Cortney Davis MSN, NP	Poetry, memoir, creative nonfiction
Meredith Wallace Kazer, MFA, PhD, APRN, FAAN	Fiction
Theresa Brown	Creative nonfiction

Table 3 Journals dedicated to the illness experience	
Journal	**Discipline**
SANA: Self-Achievement Through Creative Art	Nursing
The Intima	Medicine
Humanism Evolving through Arts and Literature (HEAL)	Medical Humanities

system or a provider. Written words, whether it is poetry, prose, nonfiction, or a creative nonfiction essay, produce a common language between patients, providers, and laypersons. The use of the written word, specifically through reflective practices, facilitate creative empathetic growth through a personal examination of personal biases, fostering sensitivity, and identify potential barriers to care such as fear, discrimination, stigma, or differences in culture.

Professional conferences are now recognizing and offering the opportunity for the nursing community to submit artwork representing an impact on the self or others. Organizations such as Sigma Theta Tau, the International Honors Society of Nursing, advertise a call for abstracts specifically for creative works of all mediums including the written word, visual (photography, video, painting, etc), knitting, quilting, or performances (dance).[33]

Creative works stretch beyond professional conferences and have long been present in the medical and nursing literature. The *Journal of the American Medical Association* and *The Lancet*, 2 of the longest running medical journals, publish and feature columns dedicated to medical themed art. The *American Journal of Nursing* hosts a column entitled "Reflections," reserved for the personal exploration essay. It is within this use of art and personal exploration where one may discover strengths, embody a lived experience, and connects the writer to the larger world in which we live.[34] There are a number of medical, nursing, and medical humanities journals dedicated to curation of expressive art focused on the illness experience (**Table 3**).

NURSING PORTRAYED IN THE POPULAR ARTS

Nurses, including those practicing in a critical care environment, are consistently portrayed on television and film. The nurse is typically cast as a female with only a few, rare exceptions. Men portrayed as nurses in popular television shows typically reinforce gender stereotypes.[35] Writers, visionaries, and producers should work together to bring storylines to life while representing the culture of nursing and cultivating an inclusive society. Similarly, nursing and medicine have long the subject of artwork (**Table 4**). The nurses depicted in artwork of the time period often reflect the uniform and the role of the nurse. Many of these works were not created by nurses and are the perception of nursing from others outside of the discipline.

Table 4 Nurses in art			
Title	**Artist**	**Year**	**Medium**
The Attentive Nurse	Jean Siméon Chardin, (French)	Probably 1738	Oil on canvas
Portrait of a Nurse	Lewis W. Hine (American, 1874–1940)	ca. 1909–1935	Photography: negative, gelatin on diacetate film

SUMMARY

There is much discussion around the art *of* nursing but it is time to spotlight the importance and the implications of art *in* nursing. Nursing and the illness experience are the subjects for many fiction, nonfiction, and poetry collections. There are stories written from the practitioner's point of view and notable literature written from the patient's perspective. Illness, mild or critical, is a human experience, one that can be uniting or dividing. A lived experience that does not spare anyone of any age, culture, background, or foreground.

In the black and white critical care realm where complexity touches systems and humans, creativity and artful expressions add the important colors of life. Articulating an event further developments of empathy in the nurse and in the person receiving care, regardless of one's own previous experience's with illness. Creative expression through self-reflection on one's own practice, narrative arts, visuals, auditory, tactile, or through a different medium may aid in the restoration of an individual's purpose and serve as a reminder as to why one chose to pursue the art of nursing.

DISCLOSURE

The author has nothing to disclose.

REFERENCES

1. Dimitroff BLJ. Journaling: a valuable tool for registered nurses. Am Nurse Today 2018;13(11):27–8.
2. Halm MA. Intensive care unit diaries, part 1: constructing illness narratives to promote recovery after critical illness. Am J Crit Care 2019;28(4):319–24.
3. Pattison N, O'Gara G, Lucas C, et al. Filling the gaps: a mixed-methods study exploring the use of patient diaries in the critical care unit. Intensive Crit Care Nurs 2019;51:27–34.
4. Chlan LL. Music therapy as a nursing intervention for patients supported by mechanical ventilation. AACN Clin Issues 2000;11(1):128–38.
5. World Health Organization. Self-care can be an effective part of national health systems. 2019. Available at: https://www.who.int/reproductivehealth/self-care-national-health-systems/en/.
6. Ruppar TM, Cooper PS, Johnson ED, et al. Self-care interventions for adults with heart failure: a systematic review and meta-analysis protocol. J Adv Nurs 2019; 75(3):676–82.
7. Association AD. Older adults: standards of medical care in diabetes. Diabetes Care 2019;42:S139–47.
8. Harrison SL, Janaudis-Ferreira T, Brooks D, et al. Self-management following an acute exacerbation of COPD: a systematic review. Chest 2015;147(3):646–61.
9. Zimbudzi E, Lo C, Misso ML, et al. Effectiveness of self-management support interventions for people with comorbid diabetes and chronic kidney disease: a systematic review and meta-analysis. Syst Rev 2018;7(1). https://doi.org/10.1186/s13643-018-0748-z.
10. Coleman EA, Roman SP, Hall KA, et al. Enhancing the care transitions intervention protocol to better address the needs of family caregivers. J Healthc Qual 2015;37(1):2–11.
11. Deci EL, Ryan RM. Hedonia, eudaimonia, and well-being: an introduction. J Happiness Stud 2008;9(1):1–11.

12. Gellera G, Thompson JW. Nicomachean ethics. Nicomachean Ethics 2017;1–97. https://doi.org/10.4324/9781912281848.
13. Costa DK, Moss M. The cost of caring: emotion, burnout, and psychological distress in critical care clinicians. Ann Am Thorac Soc 2018;15(7):787–90.
14. Moss M, Good VS, Kleinpell R, et al. The cost of caring: emotion, burnout, and psychological distress in critical care clinicians. Am J Crit Care 2006;15(4):18–20.
15. Maslow A. Toward a psychology. 2nd edition 1968.
16. Empathy. Oxford English Dictionary.
17. Treadaway C. Materiality, memory and imagination: using empathy to research creativity. 2009;42(3):231–7.
18. Bautista CA, Nydahl P, Bader MK, et al. Executive summary. J Neurosci Nurs 2019;51(4):158–61.
19. Herrup EA, Wieczorek B, Kudchadkar SR. Characteristics of postintensive care syndrome in survivors of pediatric critical illness: a systematic review. World J Crit Care Med 2017;6(2):124.
20. Society of Critical Care Medicine. Post Intensive Care Syndrome.
21. Mikkelsen ME, Jackson JC, Hopkins RO, et al. Peer support as a novel strategy to mitigate post-intensive care syndrome. AACN Adv Crit Care 2016;27(2):221–9.
22. Garrouste-Orgeas M, Flahault C, Vinatier I, et al. Effect of an ICU diary on post-traumatic stress disorder symptoms among patients receiving mechanical ventilation. JAMA 2019;322(3):229.
23. Blair KTA, Eccleston SD, Binder HM, et al. Improving the patient experience by implementing an ICU diary for those at risk of post-intensive care syndrome. J Patient Exp 2017;4(1):4–9.
24. Alligood MR. Testing Roger's theory of accelerating change. the relationships among creativity, actualization, and empathy in persons 18 to 92 years of age. West J Nurs Res 1991;13:84–96.
25. NCSBN. National Nursing Workforce Study.
26. Liu H-Y, Wang I-T, Han H-M, et al. Perceived self-efficacy of teaching for creativity among nurse faculty in Taiwan. Nurs Educ Perspect 2019;40(6):E19–21.
27. Rivosecchi RM, Kane-Gill SL, Svec S, et al. The implementation of a nonpharmacologic protocol to prevent intensive care delirium. J Crit Care 2016;31(1):206–11.
28. Galiczewski JM. Interventions for the prevention of catheter associated urinary tract infections in intensive care units: an integrative review. Intensive Crit Care Nurs 2016;32:1–11.
29. Swafford BK, Culpepper R, Dunn C. Use of a comprehensive program to reduce the incidence of hospital-acquired pressure ulcers in an intensive care unit. Am J Crit Care 2016;25(2):152–5.
30. Dubb R, Nydahl P, Hermes C, et al. Barriers and strategies for early mobilization of patients in intensive care units. Ann Am Thorac Soc 2016;13(5):724–30.
31. Gholami M, Kordestani P, Mohammadipoor F. Comparing the effects of problem-based learning and the traditional lecture method on critical thinking skills and metacognitive awareness in nursing students in a critical care nursing course ☆. Nurse Educ Today 2016;45:16–21. https://doi.org/10.1016/j.nedt.2016.06.007.
32. Green MJ, Myers K, Watson K, et al. Creativity in medical education: the value of having medical students make stuff. J Med Humanit 2016;37(4):475–83.
33. Sigma Theta Tau - call for abstracts. 2019. Available at: https://www.sigmanursing.org/connect-engage/meetings-events/convention/call-for-abstracts.
34. Osler T, Guillard I, Garcia-Fialdini A, et al. An a/r/tographic métissage: storying the self as pedagogic practice. J Writ Creat Pract 2019;12(1–2):109–29.
35. Weaver R, Ferguson C, Wilbourn M, et al. Men in nursing on television: exposing and reinforcing stereotypes. J Adv Nurs 2014;70(4):833–42.

Moving?

Make sure your subscription moves with you!

To notify us of your new address, find your **Clinics Account Number** (located on your mailing label above your name), and contact customer service at:

Email: journalscustomerservice-usa@elsevier.com

800-654-2452 (subscribers in the U.S. & Canada)
314-447-8871 (subscribers outside of the U.S. & Canada)

Fax number: 314-447-8029

Elsevier Health Sciences Division
Subscription Customer Service
3251 Riverport Lane
Maryland Heights, MO 63043

*To ensure uninterrupted delivery of your subscription, please notify us at least 4 weeks in advance of move.

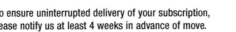

Printed and bound by CPI Group (UK) Ltd, Croydon, CR0 4YY

03/10/2024

01040481-0012